Evaluation and Management of Common Upper Extremity Disorders

A Practical Handbook

T0386309

Edited by

Rachel S. Rohde, MD
Assistant Professor of Orthopaedic Surgery
Oakland University
William Beaumont School of Medicine
Royal Oak, Michigan

Peter J. Millett, MD, MSc
Director of Shoulder Surgery
Shoulder and Sports Medicine
The Steadman Clinic
Vail, Colorado

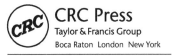

CRC Press
Taylor & Francis Group
Boca Raton London New York

CRC Press is an imprint of the
Taylor & Francis Group, an **informa** business

First published 2011 by SLACK Incorporated

Published 2024 by CRC Press
2385 NW Executive Center Drive, Suite 320, Boca Raton FL 33431

and by CRC Press
4 Park Square, Milton Park, Abingdon, Oxon, OX14 4RN

CRC Press is an imprint of Taylor & Francis Group, LLC

© 2011 Taylor & Francis Group, LLC

Library of Congress Cataloging-in-Publication Data
Evaluation and management of common upper extremity disorders : a practical handbook / edited by Rachel Rohde, Peter Millett.
    p. ; cm.
  Includes bibliographical references and index.
  Summary: "*Evaluation and Management of Common Upper Extremity Disorders: A Practical Handbook* answers the need for a comprehensive, yet concise reference that addresses practical solutions to everyday conditions that general orthopedic surgeons, and specialists alike, as well those involved with general musculoskeletal surgical and nonsurgical care, may encounter. This book provides information on how to diagnose, treat, and manage the most commonly encountered conditions of the upper extremity. Written in a bullet format, and including photos for quick, easy reference, the book contains valuable information for all levels of training and experience"--Provided by publisher.
  ISBN 9781556429491 (pbk. : alk. paper)
  1. Arm--Diseases--Treatment--Handbook, manuals, etc. 2. Arm--Wounds and injuries--Treatment--Handbooks, manuals, etc. I. Rohde, Rachel S., 1973- II. Millett, Peter J. (Peter James), 1967-
  [DNLM: 1. Upper Extremity--injuries--Handbooks. 2. Upper Extremity--pathology--Handbooks. 3. Musculoskeletal Diseases--diagnosis--Handbooks. 4. Musculoskeletal Diseases--therapy--Handbooks. WE 39]
  RC951.E88 2011
  617.5'74--dc22

                                                      2011014492

ISBN: 9781556429491 (pbk)
ISBN: 9781003524052 (ebk)

DOI: 10.1201/9781003524052

DEDICATION

To my husband, Steven, and our daughter, Sydney,
who was born during the creation of this book.

—RSR

To the medical students, residents, and fellows
I have trained and have trained with
for teaching me so much and
inspiring me to learn more.

—PJM

CONTENTS

Acknowledgments

We would like to acknowledge our contributing authors for dedicating their time, energy, and knowledge to this project. Carrie Kotlar, our Acquisitions Editor at SLACK Incorporated, brought us together to create this book. The efforts of Ms. Kotlar, John Bond, Jennifer Cahill, April Billick, and Michelle Gatt made this work possible.

—RSR

Thank you to Marilee Horan, MPH, and Rochelle Grove, who keep me organized, on time (mostly!), and moving forward with our research and academic projects.

—PJM

ABOUT THE EDITORS

Rachel S. Rohde, MD, is certified by the American Board of Orthopaedic Surgery and holds a Certificate of Added Qualifications in Hand Surgery. Currently an Assistant Professor of Orthopaedic Surgery at Oakland University William Beaumont School of Medicine, she specializes in treatment of musculoskeletal conditions of the upper extremity at William Beaumont Hospital in Royal Oak, Michigan.

Following undergraduate studies at The University of Michigan in Ann Arbor, Dr. Rohde earned her medical degree from Harvard Medical School and Massachusetts Institute of Technology. She completed an orthopedic surgery residency program and was a Visiting Instructor in orthopedic surgery at The University of Pittsburgh Medical Center. In addition, she completed a fellowship in upper extremity, hand, and microvascular surgery at Hospital for Special Surgery in New York City.

Dr. Rohde is an American Orthopaedic Association Emerging Leader and an American Society for Surgery of the Hand Young Leader. She also is involved in the American Association for Hand Surgery and is a Fellow of the American Academy of Orthopaedic Surgeons. Her research has been published in several peer-reviewed journals, and she has presented her findings at regional, national, and international meetings. Her book *Acute Management of Hand Injuries,* published by SLACK Incorporated, was released in January 2009.

Peter J. Millett, MD, MSc, is a partner at The Steadman Clinic and an internationally recognized orthopedic surgeon specializing in disorders of the shoulder and all sports-related injuries. Consistently selected as one of the "Best Doctors in America," Dr. Millett serves as a shoulder and sports medicine consultant to the country of Bermuda and has treated elite athletes from the NFL, NBA, MLB, X-Games, and the Olympics. Prior to coming to Vail, Dr. Millett held a faculty appointment at Harvard Medical School and was formerly Co-Director of the Harvard Shoulder Service and the Harvard Shoulder Fellowship.

Contributing Authors

Robert E. Boykin, MD (Chapter 12)
Department of Orthopaedic Surgery
Massachusetts General Hospital
Boston, Massachusetts

Sepp Braun, MD (Chapter 11)
Department of Orthopaedic Sports Medicine
Technische Universität München
Klinikum rechts der Isar
Munich, Germany

Michael Darowish, MD (Chapter 7)
Assistant Professor
Department of Orthopedic Surgery
Milton S. Hershey Medical Center
Penn State College of Medicine
Hershey, Pennsylvania

Christopher B. Dewing, MD (Chapter 9)
Lieutenant Commander, MC, USN
Assistant Director Sports Surgery
Department of Orthopedic Surgery
Naval Medical Center San Diego
San Diego, California

Florian Elser, MD (Chapter 11)
Hessingpark-Clinic
Sportsmedicine and Traumatology
Augsburg, Germany

David C. Gerhardt, MD (Chapter 6)
Department of Orthopaedic Surgery
University of Colorado—Denver
Denver, Colorado

Reuben Gobezie, MD (Chapter 10)
Chief, Division of Shoulder and Elbow Surgery
Case Western Reserve University/
University Hospitals of Cleveland
Cleveland, Ohio

Danny P. Goel, MD, FRCSC (Chapter 14)
Burnaby, British Columbia

Robert R. L. Gray, MD (Chapter 5)
Assistant Professor of Orthopaedic Surgery
Division of Hand Surgery
University of Miami Miller School of Medicine
Miami, Florida

James J. Guerra, MD, FACS (Chapter 10)
Head Team Physician
Florida Gulf Coast University
Fort Myers, Florida
Ave Maria University
Ave Maria, Florida

Hinrich J. D. Heuer (Chapters 10, 12, 13)
The Steadman Clinic and
Steadman Philippon Research Institute
Vail, Colorado

Christopher J. Lenarz, MD (Chapter 10)
Department of Orthopaedic Surgery
Division of Shoulder and Elbow
Case Western Reserve University School of Medicine
Cleveland, Ohio

Kimberly Mezera, MD (Chapter 4)
Associate Professor
Medical Director
Orthopaedic Surgery Clinic and Upper Extremity Services
UT Southwestern Medical Center
Dallas, Texas

Ryan G. Miyamoto, MD (Chapter 8)
Orthopaedic Surgeon
Fair Oaks Orthopaedics
Fair Oaks Hospital
Fairfax, Virginia

Charles J. Petit, MD (Chapter 9)
Private Practice
Cascade Orthopedics and Sports Medicine, PC
The Dalles, Oregon

Brent A. Ponce, MD (Chapter 13)
Assistant Professor
University of Alabama at Birmingham
Birmingham, Alabama

James R. Romanowski, MD (Chapter 14)
Director
The Ohio Shoulder Institute
Columbus, Ohio

Gregory V. Sobol, MD (Chapter 3)
Hand and Upper Extremity Surgery
William Beaumont Hospital
Royal Oak, Michigan

Peter Tang, MD, MPH (Chapter 1)
Assistant Professor of Clinical Orthopaedic Surgery
New York Presbyterian Hospital
Columbia University Medical Center
New York, New York

Walter W. Virkus, MD (Chapter 5)
Associate Professor
Residency Program Director
Department of Orthopedic Surgery
Rush University Medical Center
Chicago, Illinois

Jon J. P. Warner, MD (Chapter 14)
Chief, The Harvard Shoulder Service
Professor of Orthopaedic Surgery
Massachusetts General Hospital
Harvard Medical School
Boston, Massachusetts

Trent J. Wilson, MD (Chapter 13)
Orthopaedic Surgery Resident
University of Alabama at Birmingham
Birmingham, Alabama

Jennifer Moriatis Wolf, MD (Chapter 6)
Associate Professor
Orthopaedic Surgery
New England Musculoskeletal Institute
University of Connecticut Medical Center
Farmington, Connecticut

of pediatric trigger thumb is beyond the scope of this text.

ADDITIONAL TESTING OR IMAGING

- Additional testing is not performed routinely and usually is not needed to make the diagnosis.
- Radiographs can be considered to evaluate for arthritis if there is decreased motion of the finger.
- Special testing for some of the associated medical conditions can be considered if suspected.

TREATMENT OPTIONS: NONOPERATIVE

- **Activity modification** may be beneficial in early cases. However, it has not been established that there is a direct link between activity and trigger finger. Advising patients to try to avoid activities that aggravate their symptoms is reasonable. This author tells patients to refrain from heavy gripping activities such as hammering.
- **Splinting** may be beneficial in early cases. The splints should hold the MCP joint in neutral extension or in 10 to 15 degrees of flexion. In order to be effective, the splint must be worn for at least 4 months. This author rarely recommends this option and prescribes it if the patient defers other interventions or complains of significant pain.
- **Nonsteroidal anti-inflammatory drugs** (NSAIDs) can be of benefit.
- **Steroid injections** have a reported rate of effectiveness from 42% to as high as 92% with as many as 3 injections.[1,3,5-8] Efficacy is diminished in patients with diabetes, a long duration of symptoms, and more injections. **Patients with diabetes should be warned that after steroid injections, hyperglycemia**

may last for 5 days.[9] Other side effects include fat atrophy and hypopigmentation. Tendon rupture has been described.

- Regarding steroid selection, one prospective, randomized study evaluated dexamethasone versus triamcinolone and found that triamcinolone was more effective at 6 weeks, but that they demonstrated equal efficacy at 3 months.[10] In another study, comparison of 1, 2, or 3 injections before surgical release, immediate surgical release, and immediate percutaneous release showed the most cost-effective treatment algorithm to be 2 steroid injections followed by surgical release if needed.[11]

TREATMENT OPTIONS: OPERATIVE

Open surgery entails complete release of the A1 pulley. If this fails to relieve the triggering, the ulnar slip of the flexor digitorum superficialis (FDS) tendon may be excised to decrease the total volume of the flexor tendons.

Special Cases

Treatment of the pediatric trigger finger, which occurs much less frequently than the trigger thumb, also involves A1 pulley release and FDS slip excision.[12] Despite this treatment, clicking may persist in the pediatric trigger finger and may be caused by a problem located more distally involving abnormal tendon anatomy or the decussation between the FDS and flexor digitorum profundus (FDP).

In patients with rheumatoid arthritis, it is not advisable to release the A1 pulley because it may lead to ulnar drift of the fingers; instead, the recommended treatment is tenosynovectomy, excision of rheumatoid nodules, resection of the ulnar slip of the FDS, and preservation of the A1 pulley.

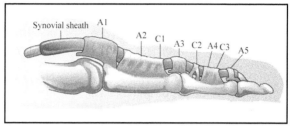

Figure 1-1. Illustration of the flexor tendon pulley system. (Adapted from Doyle JR. Hand. In: Doyle JR, Botte MJ, eds. *Surgical Anatomy of the Hand & Upper Extremity.* Philadelphia, PA: Lippincott Williams and Wilkins; 2003:600.)

SURGICAL ANATOMY

- Immediately volar to the A1 pulley is the FDS; deep to the FDS lies the FDP.
- Proximal to the A1 pulley may be a thin layer of palmar pulley and distal to it, the A2 pulley (Figure 1-1). Some anatomy references locate the C1 pulley to be between the A1 and A2; anatomical studies have shown that there is a 50% incidence of continuity between the A1 and A2 pulleys.[13]
- Bordering the A1 pulley are the radial and ulnar digital nerves; deep to the nerves at this level are the digital arteries. In the thumb, the **radial digital nerve** is most at risk because it travels from ulnar to radial **across the A1 pulley** and has been found to be 1.19 mm deep to the dermis, so it can be inadvertently transected with a deep skin incision.

PROCEDURES

Open release will be described. Percutaneous needle release and pediatric trigger release are beyond the scope of this book.

- The patient is positioned supine on the operating room table with the upper extremity on a hand table. A tourniquet is applied to the forearm or arm and the hand is prepped and draped sterilely. Either local anesthesia or a Bier block with or without intravenous sedation can be used; use of local anesthesia without, or with minimal, sedation allows the patient to flex and extend the digit actively after pulley release to confirm complete release.
- The incision can be oblique, transverse, or longitudinal (Figure 1-2). Most surgeons will try to incorporate the local palmar flexion creases. When addressing the thumb, placing the incision in the MCP flexion crease is ideal. An oblique extension of the distal palmar flexion crease is ideal for the index finger. In the long finger, the radial part of the distal palmar flexion crease is centered over the A1 pulley. Lastly, the distal palmar flexion crease at the ring and small fingers will be at the proximal extent of the A1 pulley. If multiple fingers are to be released, one long transverse incision can be made across the palm or multiple short incisions can be used.
- After anesthesia administration, the extremity is exsanguinated and the tourniquet (if used) is inflated. The skin and dermis are incised. Particular care is taken in the thumb to prevent injury to the superficially located radial digital nerve.
- Scissors are used to dissect bluntly down to the A1 pulley (Figure 1-3). In the thumb, it is advisable to identify the radial and ulnar digital nerves. In the fingers, one should try to identify the digital nerves; however, if they are not easily found, to prevent iatrogenic injury, the soft tissue on the radial and ulnar sides of the pulley simply are retracted. With appropriate retraction and a clear view of the A1 pulley the nerves should be safe. Distal and proximal skin flaps above the flexor sheath are developed to create a working space.

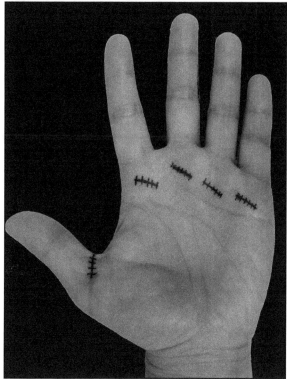

Figure 1-2. Author's preferred incisions for A1 pulley releases of all digits. The thumb metacarpophalangeal joint flexion crease is a reliable location for incision. This author uses an oblique incision volar to metacarpophalangeal joints and tries to incorporate palmar flexion creases for trigger release of the fingers. Other options for the fingers include longitudinal and transverse incisions. If all fingers are being released, the incision may be one continuous transverse incision or multiple small incisions.

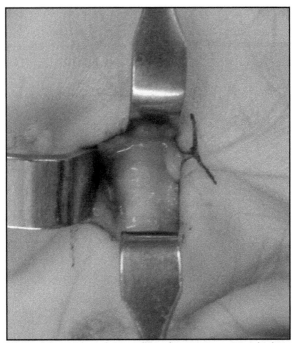

Figure 1-3. Thickened A1 pulley after exposure in right long finger (top is distal and bottom is proximal).

- When the A1 pulley is identified clearly, it is incised; care is taken not to injure the flexor tendons deep to the pulley. The A1 pulley of the trigger finger is often very thick. The A1 pulley is approximately 1 cm long and may be even shorter; this should be kept in mind so that the A2 pulley, sometimes in continuity with the A1 pulley, is preserved.
- One useful technique to help identify the proximal extent of the A2 pulley is to perform the "snap" test. Following A1 pulley release, a hemostat with the

tip pointed volarly is placed under the A2 pulley. The tip is pushed against the pulley and is withdrawn proximally. The hemostat will snap against the proximal end of the A2 pulley; if there is still pulley holding the hemostat, it is either remaining A1 pulley, which should be released, or C1 pulley, which can be released.

- In the thumb, the pulley distal to A1 is the oblique pulley.
- Once the A1 pulley is released, the tendons can be pulled out of the incision and evaluated for fraying. Frayed ends may be débrided, but this probably will not affect the outcome.
- Identified nerves should be inspected for any injury.
- The tourniquet is released and the wound irrigated. A bipolar electrocautery is used to obtain hemostasis, keeping in mind the location of the nerves so as not to cause inadvertent injury.
- The skin is closed with the surgeon's choice of suture and fashion; this author uses 4-0 nylon in a horizontal mattress. A sterile soft dressing is applied.

REHABILITATION

- Immediately after surgery, the patient is encouraged to elevate the extremity and work on full extension and flexion of all the fingers.
- Occupational hand therapy usually is not necessary but may be needed when multiple trigger fingers are released or if there is decreased motion at the 2-week postoperative visit.

OUTCOMES

- Open release: Surgical treatment has been found to be 97% effective in patients.[14]
- Open versus percutaneous release: Both procedures have been found to be equally successful.[15]

POTENTIAL COMPLICATIONS

- Digital nerve injury (although injury to digital nerves has not been reported with percutaneous release, some authors do not recommend this technique for the index finger or thumb because of the proximity of the nerves[16])
- Digital artery injury
- A2 pulley injury
- Bowstringing
- Recurrence of symptoms
- Scar sensitivity
- Sympathetic dystrophy
- Shower emboli and digital necrosis (there is one reported case of a steroid injection causing these complications, which resolved[17]; it is hypothesized that the injection was intra-arterial)

DE QUERVAIN'S TENOSYNOVITIS

MECHANISM OF INJURY/ PATHOPHYSIOLOGY

De Quervain's disease is caused by attritional forces secondary to friction that cause swelling and thickening of the extensor retinaculum of the first dorsal compartment. This leads to restricted gliding of the abductor pollicis longus (APL) and the extensor pollicis brevis (EPB). The condition affects women more frequently than it does men. The patient is commonly older than 40 years of age, except when the process affects pregnant and lactating women. The etiology is not completely clear, but the following theories have been offered to explain it:

- Repetitive lifting and manipulation
- Trauma
- Increased frictional forces
- Anatomic abnormality
- Biomechanical compression
- Repetitive microtrauma
- Inflammatory disease
- Increased volume states, such as during pregnancy

KEY HISTORY POINTS

- Patients present with insidious onset of radial-sided wrist pain.
- The pain is exacerbated by lifting objects with the wrist in neutral rotation as well as activities that require prolonged thumb extension.
- Rarely, patients report triggering with thumb extension or abduction.[18]

KEY EXAMINATION POINTS

- There is swelling and tenderness to palpation at the first dorsal compartment. This author makes the diagnosis based solely on age, history, swelling, and tenderness.
- There may be a firm nodule in the area, representing thickening of the compartment.
- The classic pathognomic maneuver is Finkelstein's test, which entails grasping the patient's thumb and quickly deviating the hand and wrist ulnarly. If this reproduces the pain, the test is considered positive.
- The Eichoff maneuver entails having the patient clench the thumb in a fist and then briskly deviating the wrist ulnarly.
- Pain may be elicited with resisted thumb MCP joint extension, which isolates the EPB.
- The differential for pain on the radial side of the wrist also includes intersection syndrome (tenderness 4 to 5 cm proximal to the wrist joint over the second dorsal compartment), radial styloid and scaphoid fracture (history of trauma and positive radiographs), carpometacarpal (CMC) joint arthritis or synovitis (CMC tenderness), and radial neuritis (Tinel's sign).

ADDITIONAL TESTING OR IMAGING

- **Radiographs** are not needed to make the diagnosis but may be helpful to exclude fracture diagnoses in the setting of trauma.
- **Magnetic resonance imaging and ultrasound** are of no benefit in making the diagnosis.

TREATMENT OPTIONS: NONOPERATIVE

- **Activity modification** is recommended to minimize the activities that exacerbate the condition. This author suggests minimizing activities that involve prolonged thumb extension and wrist radial deviation. This may prove difficult for new mothers picking up a child and supporting the child's head.

- **Thumb spica splints** to rest the compartment and its tendons can be helpful. Lane and colleagues found splinting and NSAIDs effective in 88% of patients with minimal symptoms but only 32% effective when the symptoms were moderate to severe.[19] Weiss and associates evaluated steroid injection alone, splinting alone, and in combination; they reported 67% improvement with injection alone, 57% improvement with both injection and splinting, and 19% improvement with splinting alone.[20] They recommended injection alone and not splinting. Despite this study, this author prescribes a splint.

- **NSAIDs** can be a treatment option. This author recommends NSAIDs if the symptoms are mild or if the patient declines a steroid injection. One study found no benefit when nimesulide, a selective cyclooxygenase-2 inhibitor, was given with a steroid injection.[21]

- **Steroid injection** has a success rate ranging from 62% to 93%.[22] Failure of injection has been purported to be due to failure to deliver the steroid into the separate EPB compartment.[23] Complications of the injection are the same as for trigger finger.

TREATMENT OPTIONS: OPERATIVE

The goal of operative treatment is complete release of the first dorsal compartment including any individual compartments of multiple slips of the APL or EPB.

SURGICAL ANATOMY

- The first dorsal compartment is approximately 2 cm long and is located on the radial side of the distal radius proximal to the radiocarpal joint.
- The APL tendon is more volar and inserts on the base of the first metacarpal, while the EPB tendon is more dorsal and inserts on the base of the proximal phalanx of the thumb.
- The first dorsal compartment has an additional septum in 60% of patients with de Quervain's tenosynovitis, and the APL consists of multiple tendons in 76% of these patients.[24] The EPB tendon also can have multiple slips.

PROCEDURES

- The patient is positioned supinely with the operative extremity on a hand table. A forearm or upper arm tourniquet is applied and the arm is prepared and draped sterilely. Local anesthesia with or without intravenous sedation is used.
- The incision can be longitudinal, transverse, oblique, or chevron (Figure 1-4).
- After the skin is incised, scissors are used to dissect to the first compartment, while branches of the superficial radial nerve are retracted and preserved.
- Skin flaps are elevated.
- The APL, EPB, and all slips of the tendons are identified proximal to entering the compartment and

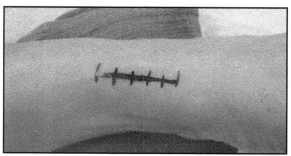

Figure 1-4. Skin incision for first dorsal compartment release in a left wrist (right is distal and left is proximal).

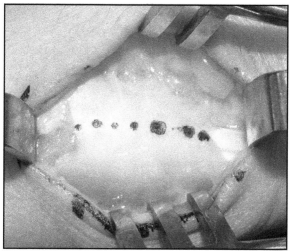

Figure 1-5. The dotted line shows the proposed dorsally located incision of the compartment. Proximal to the compartment (left), there is tenosynovitis of the tendons.

distal to the compartment as they exit (Figure 1-5). This identification decreases the probability of failing to release a subcompartment.

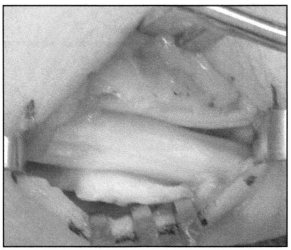

Figure 1-6. After compartment release.

- An incision is made on the dorsal aspect of the first dorsal compartment; a volar flap is left intact to prevent volar subluxation of the tendons[25] (Figures 1-6 and 1-7).
- Any septations dividing the compartment into sub-compartments are released. All slips of the tendons are released.
- The thumb and wrist are ranged to evaluate for volar subluxation of the tendons (Figure 1-8).
- If excessive subluxation is concerning, this author sutures the volar flap to the subcutaneous fat of the volar skin flap, protecting any branches of the superficial radial nerve.
- Repairing the compartment is not recommended.
- The tourniquet is released, the wound is irrigated, and hemostasis is obtained.
- The skin is closed and a sterile dressing and thumb spica splint are applied.

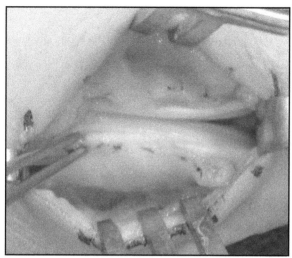

Figure 1-7. Volar flap of the compartment being held by forceps.

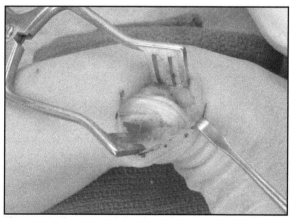

Figure 1-8. The wrist and thumb are flexed to evaluate for volar tendon subluxation, which is not present as shown in the picture.

REHABILITATION

- Therapy usually is needed only in cases of significant stiffness.
- All patients are taught scar massage.

OUTCOMES

- The success rate of surgical release is 91% or greater.[26-30]

POTENTIAL COMPLICATIONS

- Injury to branches of the superficial radial nerve
- Incomplete release (most commonly of the EPB)
- Volar tendon subluxation
- Recurrence of pain
- Scar sensitivity
- Reflex sympathetic dystrophy

REFERENCES

1. Fleisch SB, Spindler KP, Lee DH. Corticosteroid injections in the treatment of trigger finger: a level I and II systematic review. *J Am Acad Orthop Surg.* 2007;15:166-171.
2. Sampson SP, Badalamente MA, Hurst LC, Seidman J. Pathobiology of the human A1 pulley in trigger finger. *J Hand Surg Am.* 1991;16:714-721.
3. Saldana MJ. Trigger digits: diagnosis and treatment. *J Am Acad Orthop Surg.* 2001;9:246-252.
4. Ryzewicz M, Wolf JM. Trigger digits: principles, management, and complications. *J Hand Surg Am.* 2006;31(1): 135-146.
5. Lambert MA, Morton RJ, Sloan JP. Controlled study of the use of local steroid injection in the treatment of trigger finger and thumb. *J Hand Surg Br.* 1992;17:69-70.

6. Murphy D, Failla JM, Koniuch MP. Steroid versus placebo injection for trigger finger. *J Hand Surg Am.* 1995;20: 628-631.

7. Taras JS, Raphael JS, Pan WT, Movagharnia F, Sotereanos DG. Corticosteroid injections for trigger digits: is intrasheath injection necessary? *J Hand Surg Am.* 1998;23:717-722.

8. Maneerit J, Sriworakun C, Budhraja N, Nagavajara P. Trigger thumb: results of a prospective randomized study of percutaneous release with steroid injection versus steroid injection alone. *J Hand Surg Br.* 2003;28:586-589.

9. Wang AA, Hutchinson DT. The effect of corticosteroid injection for trigger finger on blood glucose level in diabetic patients. *J Hand Surg Am.* 2006;31:979-981.

10. Ring D, Lozano-Calderon S, Shin R, Bastian P, Mudgal C, Jupiter J. A prospective randomized controlled trial of injection of dexamethasone versus triamcinolone for idiopathic trigger finger. *J Hand Surg Am.* 2008;33:516-522.

11. Kerrigan CL, Stanwix MG. Using evidence to minimize the cost of trigger finger care. *J Hand Surg Am.* 2009;34: 997-1005.

12. Bae DS, Sodha S, Waters PM. Surgical treatment of the pediatric trigger finger. *J Hand Surg Am.* 2007;32:1043-1047.

13. Lin GT, Amadio PC, An KN, Cooney WP. Functional anatomy of the human digital flexor pulley system. *J Hand Surg Am.* 1989;14:949-956.

14. Turowski GA, Zdankiewicz PD, Thomson JG. The results of surgical treatment of trigger finger. *J Hand Surg Am.* 1997;22:145-149.

15. Gilberts ECAM, Beekman WH, Stevens HJPD, Wereldsma JCJ. Prospective randomized trial of open versus percutaneous surgery for trigger digits. *J Hand Surg Am.* 2001;26:497-500.

16. Pope DF, Wolfe SW. Safety and efficacy of percutaneous trigger finger release. *J Hand Surg Am.* 1995;20: 280-283.

17. Park J, Dumanian GA. Shower emboli and digital necrosis after a single corticosteroid injection for trigger thumb: case report. *J Hand Surg Am.* 2009;34:313-316.

18. Alberton GM, High WA, Shin AY, Bishop AT. Extensor triggering in de Quervain's stenosing tenosynovitis. *J Hand Surg Am.* 1999;24:1311-1314.

19. Lane LB, Boretz RS, Stuchin SA. Treatment of de Quervain's disease: role of conservative management. *J Hand Surg Br.* 2001;26:258-260.

20. Weiss AP, Akelman E, Tabatabai M. Treatment of de Quervain's disease. *J Hand Surg Am.* 1994;19:595-598.

21. Jirarattanaphochai K, Saengnipanthkul S, Vipulakorn K, Jianmongkol S, Chatusparisute P, Jung S. Treatment of de Quervain disease with triamcinolone injection with or without nimesulide. A randomized, double-blind, placebo-controlled trial. *J Bone Joint Surg Am.* 2004;86:2700-2706.

22. Ilyas AM. Nonsurgical treatment for de Quervain's tenosynovitis. *J Hand Surg Am.* 2009;34(5):928-929.

23. Zingas C, Failla JM, Holsbeeck MV. Injection accuracy and clinical relief of de Quervain's tendinitis. *J Hand Surg Am.* 1998;23:89-96.

24. Bahm J, Szabo Z, Foucher G. The anatomy of de Quervain's syndrome: a study of operative findings. *Int Orthop.* 1995;19:209-211.

25. Burton RI, Littler JW. Tendon entrapment syndrome of first extensor compartment (de Quervain's disorder). *Curr Probl Surg.* 1975;12:32-34.

26. Finkelstein H. Stenosing tendovaginitis at the radial styloid process. *J Bone Joint Surg Am.* 1930;12:509-540.

27. Lapidus PW, Fenton R. Stenosing tenovaginitis at the wrist and fingers: report of 423 cases in 369 patients with 354 operations. *AMA Arch Surg.* 1952;64:475-487.

28. Ta KT, Eidelman D, Thomson JG. Patient satisfaction and outcomes of surgery for de Quervain's tenosynovitis. *J Hand Surg Am.* 1999;24:1071-1077.

29. Zarin M, Ahmad I. Surgical treatment of de Quervain's disease. *J Coll Physicians Surg Pak.* 2003;13:157-158.

30. Gundes H, Tosun B. Longitudinal incision in surgical release of De Quervain disease. *Tech Hand Up Extrem Surg.* 2005;9:149-152.

Relevant Review Articles

Ilyas AM. Nonsurgical treatment for de Quervain's tenosynovitis. *J Hand Surg Am.* 2009;34(5):928-929.

Ryzewicz M, Wolf JM. Trigger digits: principles, management, and complications. *J Hand Surg Am.* 2006;31(1):135-146.

CHAPTER 2 | CARPAL TUNNEL SYNDROME

Rachel S. Rohde, MD

Mechanism of Injury/ Pathophysiology

Carpal tunnel syndrome, or median nerve compression at the wrist, is an ischemic insult to the nerve caused by increased contents within the canal or external compressive factors that decrease the volume of the canal. Some of the more common etiologies include the following:

Trauma

- Acute hemorrhage from a forearm, wrist, or hand injury
- Direct compression by carpal dislocation or distal radius fracture
- High-pressure injection injury
- Compartment syndrome (increased pressure)

Medical Conditions

- Diabetes
- Hypothyroidism
- Rheumatoid arthritis
- Renal failure
- Amyloidosis
- Alcoholism

Rohde RS, Millett PJ, eds.
*Evaluation and Management
of Common Upper Extremity Disorders:
A Practical Handbook* (pp 21-34).
© 2011 Taylor & Francis Group.

- Drug toxicity
- Obesity
- Pregnancy (20% to 45%)

Anatomic Variants, Masses, and Other Space-Occupying Lesions

- Persistent median artery or other anatomic variants
- Lumbrical muscle bellies, ganglion cyst, or other mass within carpal canal
- Infection (abscess)

Environmental/Occupational

- Vibratory tool use

Idiopathic

- Most common cause, predominantly in women, with minimal inflammation noted in tenosynovium

KEY HISTORY POINTS

- Symptoms include numbness, tingling, or burning sensation in the median nerve distribution.
- Nighttime symptoms are common and might resolve with "shaking out" the hands.
- Holding a phone, newspaper, or steering wheel can exacerbate symptoms.
- Patients might complain of "clumsiness" or loss of dexterity, loss of strength, and dropping objects.

KEY EXAMINATION POINTS

As with other upper extremity conditions, evaluation from the neck to the fingertips is suggested. Examination findings commonly observed in carpal tunnel syndrome can include the following:

- Thenar muscle atrophy, which suggests severe and/or chronic nerve compression
- Skin dryness, unusual texture, or cold intolerance (can indicate median nerve sympathetic dysfunction)
- Weakness of thumb abduction graded on a 0-to-5 scale (grip and pinch strength measurements are helpful but not specific for measuring median-innervated thenar muscle strength)
- Decreased sensibility in the thumb and index, long, and ring fingers (if available, Semmes-Weinstein monofilaments are more sensitive than 2-point discrimination)
- Positive Tinel's sign (percussion of the median nerve at the wrist sends "shock" sensation in the median nerve distribution)
- Positive Phalen's test (flex the wrists for 60 seconds; a "positive" test elicits median nerve distribution numbness and tingling)
- Positive median nerve compression, or Durkin's, test (manual pressure on the median nerve for 30 seconds elicits median nerve distribution numbness and tingling)

ADDITIONAL TESTING OR IMAGING

- **Nerve conduction study/electromyography** (EMG) measures and compares the conduction velocities of the nerve proximal and distal to the carpal tunnel. It is important that this testing be performed accurately; even changes in the patient's skin temperature can alter the results. General guidelines for interpreting these tests include the following:
  - □ Motor latency greater than 4.5 ms suggests median nerve compression.

- □ Sensory latency greater than 3.5 ms suggests median nerve compression.
- □ Muscle changes on EMG (eg, fibrillation potentials, decreased motor unit recruitment) suggest chronic and/or severe nerve compression.
- □ The sensitivity of this testing has been demonstrated to be around 66% and the specificity approximately 95%. Increased latencies do not absolutely mean the patient has median nerve compression, and a normal test does not exclude the possibility of carpal tunnel syndrome.
- □ Nerve conduction study or EMG is quite useful in differentiating peripheral neuropathies from more proximal nerve compression, such as cervical nerve root compression, and polyneuropathy.
- **Radiographs** of the wrist, including a carpal tunnel view, might be beneficial in identifying wrist pathology, including potential radio-opaque masses protruding into the carpal canal. For example, an unrecognized remote carpal injury can lead to median nerve compression by the lunate. However, whether radiographs are necessary with no history of wrist injury is debatable.
- **Magnetic resonance imaging and ultrasound** have been suggested to be useful, but are probably not necessary in most situations, as carpal tunnel syndrome is primarily a clinical diagnosis.
- **Laboratory tests** to evaluate for diabetes, thyroid function, or vitamin deficiency can be considered on a case-by-case basis.

TREATMENT OPTIONS: NONOPERATIVE

- **Splints** immobilizing the wrist in neutral can be effective when worn at night.

- **Steroid injection** into the carpal canal has been shown to improve symptoms in 76% of patients at 6 weeks, however, only 22% of these patients remained symptom-free at 1 year.[1] Steroid injections are most likely to help patients who have had mild symptoms for less than 1 year, normal sensory testing, and mild (if any) nerve conduction study abnormality.
    - Warn diabetic patients that transient hyperglycemia can occur for 5 days following steroid injection.
    - There is no absolute contraindication to injection in the third trimester of pregnancy or during breastfeeding, but it is advised to check with the patient's obstetrician.
- **Oral agents**
    - Nonsteroidal anti-inflammatory drugs, diuretics, and vitamin B6 have not been shown by randomized, controlled trials to be effective at alleviating symptoms.
    - Oral steroids have been shown to have short-term benefits; however, long-term effects were not studied and this treatment involves potential side effects and risks of systemic steroids.
- Ultrasound and other therapeutic endeavors have not been investigated well enough scientifically to prove that they improve symptoms. Data either are lacking or are contradictory.

TREATMENT OPTIONS: OPERATIVE

Surgical treatment for carpal tunnel syndrome involves complete transection of the transverse carpal ligament (TCL). Whether performed using open, mini-open, or endoscopic technique, the primary goal is to relieve pressure on the median nerve.

- Tenosynovectomy, internal neurolysis, and epineurotomy are not performed routinely.
- Reconstruction of the TCL is not necessary.

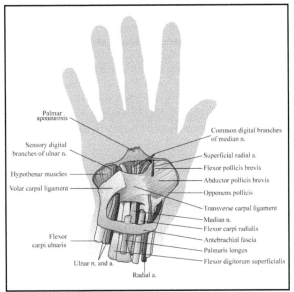

Figure 2-1. Through the carpal canal traverse 9 flexor tendons and the median nerve; overlying all of these structures is the transverse carpal ligament.

SURGICAL ANATOMY

- Within the carpal canal, the median nerve and 9 flexor tendons traverse to the digits. The canal borders are the carpal bones dorsally, radially, and ulnarly and the TCL palmarly (Figure 2-1).
- The distal aspect of the TCL extends from the hook of the hamate ulnarly to the trapezial ridge radially.
- The proximal aspect of the TCL extends from the pisiform ulnarly to the scaphoid tubercle radially. This generally is considered to be at the distal wrist crease.
- The deep distal forearm fascia might contribute to nerve compression and is released also.

Recurrent Motor Branch of Median Nerve

- Innervates most thenar muscles (opponens pollicis, abductor pollicis brevis, and half of flexor pollicis brevis)
- Usually arises from the radial side of the median nerve distal to the TCL
- Variations include the following:
  - Arising beneath the TCL but exiting distal to the ligament ("subligamentous")
  - Arising beneath and exiting through the TCL ("transligamentous") (Figure 2-2)
  - Arising and exiting proximal to the TCL
  - Arising from the ulnar side of the median nerve

Palmar Cutaneous Branch of Median Nerve

- Supplies sensation to the thenar area of the palm
- Arises from the median nerve 5 to 8.5 cm proximal to the distal wrist crease and penetrates the distal forearm fascia 1 to 4.5 cm proximal to the crease, usually coursing between flexor carpi radialis and palmaris longus (if present)
- Can cause loss of sensation and/or painful neuroma when transected

PROCEDURES

Open or limited-open carpal tunnel release is described. Endoscopic carpal tunnel release is beyond the scope of this text.

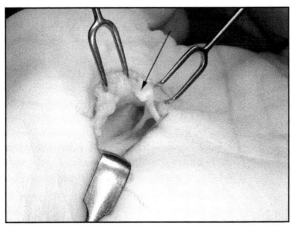

Figure 2-2. Transligamentous recurrent motor branch of median nerve; it is important to recognize and protect this branch.

- A forearm or upper arm tourniquet is used; the prepared site should allow for extension of the incision to include exposure of the distal forearm fascia if necessary.
- An incision is marked along the proximal palm in line with the fourth metacarpal. This also can be identified using the ulnar border of the flexed ring finger or the radial border of the extended ring finger (Figure 2-3). If possible, incising in a natural crease tends to produce a more cosmetic scar.
- Planned extension of this incision proximal to the distal wrist crease is curved ulnarly to avoid injury to the palmar cutaneous branch.
- Local or regional anesthesia is administered.
- The limb is exsanguinated and the tourniquet inflated.
- The skin is incised and the soft tissues dissected gently to reveal the palmar aponeurosis; these

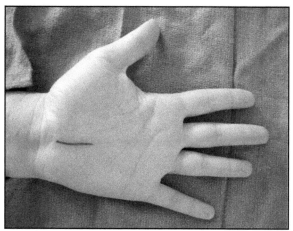

Figure 2-3. A mini-open incision allows visualization of the transverse carpal ligament; the proximal soft tissues will need to be retracted away from the palm to visualize and release the distal forearm fascia subcutaneously.

fibers are longitudinally oriented, or parallel to the incision.

- Retraction with a small self-retaining retractor helps one visualize the palmar aponeurosis, which then is incised longitudinally.

- The fibers of the TCL are oriented transversely, or perpendicular to the incision. Some of the ligament might be obscured by palmaris brevis muscle tissue. This can be cleared gently with transverse motions of a Freer or a blade held perpendicular to the fibers.

- The TCL is incised longitudinally from the most distal aspect to the most proximal aspect under direct visualization. Care is taken to release completely distally without damaging the palmar arch or common digital nerves. Identification of the perineural

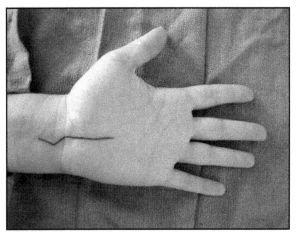

Figure 2-4. A standard open incision extends proximal to the wrist crease. The incision generally is curved ulnarly to avoid the palmar cutaneous branch of the median nerve.

and perivascular fat just past the distal edge of the TCL usually demonstrates distal release.

- The distal forearm fascia can be released a few different ways. Each of these methods requires certainty that the tissues volar and dorsal to the fascia are cleared of adherent tendon, nerve, and skin.
    - ☐ The incision can be extended proximally slightly ulnarly so that the forearm fascia can be divided under direct visualization (Figure 2-4).
    - ☐ The soft tissues can be cleared from the fascia under direct visualization (from inside the wound) subcutaneously and fascial release completed with fine, sharp tenotomy scissors (Figure 2-5).
    - ☐ Some surgeons use a mini-open assistive device instead of tenotomy scissors; proper training in these methods is recommended prior to use.

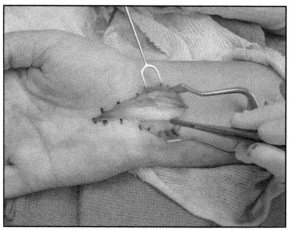

Figure 2-5. Exposure of the transverse carpal ligament and the distal forearm fascia allows median nerve release under direct visualization.

□ Always ensure complete visualization of structures before incising; **never cut what you cannot see.**

- Verify location and continuity of the recurrent motor branch; if it has been transected, it is better repaired **immediately** by a surgeon well trained in nerve repair techniques.
- Tourniquet release can demonstrate hyperemia of the compressed nerve and can be used to assess vascularity.
- The wound is irrigated and hemostasis achieved prior to closure with chosen sutures.
- The wound is dressed with sterile dressings. Wrist immobilization, although preferred by some surgeons, has not been shown to be beneficial.[2]

REHABILITATION

- Active range of motion, particularly of the digits, is encouraged following surgery.
- Some patients benefit from a short course of hand therapy, particularly if edema, stiffness, pillar pain, and scar management are issues.

OUTCOMES

- **Surgical versus nonsurgical treatment.** Although corticosteroid injection can relieve symptoms, at least temporarily, surgical treatment has been shown to be more effective than any nonsurgical treatment at 5 months[3] and 1 year.[4]
- **Open versus endoscopic carpal tunnel release.** Endoscopic carpal tunnel release has been shown to be associated with a 2- to 3-week earlier return to work.[5,6] No differences have been noted in outcomes at 3 months,[7] but there was a 5% revision rate in those who underwent endoscopic release, creating less patient satisfaction.
- **Bilateral carpal tunnel release.** The theoretical advantage of having both carpal tunnels released simultaneously is earlier return to work. Prospective randomized trials have not investigated simultaneous versus staged carpal tunnel releases.

POTENTIAL COMPLICATIONS[8]

- Incomplete release with persistent symptoms (most common complication of endoscopic carpal tunnel release)
- Median nerve motor branch injury
- Median nerve palmar cutaneous branch injury
- Superficial palmar arch laceration

- Pillar pain (25%, usually resolves within 3 months, most common complication of open carpal tunnel release)
- Hypertrophic scar
- Tendon adhesions and stiffness
- Hematoma
- Infection
- Recurrence (7% to 20%[9])

REFERENCES

1. Gelberman RH, Aronson D, Weisman MH. Carpal tunnel syndrome: results of a prospective trial of steroid injection and splinting. *J Bone Joint Surg Am.* 1980;62:1181-1184.
2. Cook AC, Szabo RM, Birkholz SW, King EF. Early mobilization following carpal tunnel release. A prospective randomized study. *J Hand Surg Br.* 1995;20:228-230.
3. Hui AC, Wong S, Leung CH, et al. A randomized controlled trial of surgery vs steroid injection for carpal tunnel syndrome. *Neurology.* 2005;64:2074-2078.
4. Ly-Pen D, Andréu JL, de Blas G, Sánchez-Olaso A, Millán I. Surgical decompression versus local steroid injection in carpal tunnel syndrome: a one-year, prospective, randomized, open, controlled clinical trial. *Arthritis Rheum.* 2005;52:612-619.
5. Brown RA, Gelberman RH, Seiler JG, et al. Carpal tunnel release: a prospective, randomized assessment of open and endoscopic methods. *J Bone Joint Surg Am.* 1993;75:1265-1275.
6. Trumble TE, Diao E, Abrams RA, Gilbert-Anderson MM. Single-portal endoscopic carpal tunnel release compared with open release: a prospective, randomized trial. *J Bone Joint Surg Am.* 2002;84:1107-1115.
7. Macdermid JC, Richards RS, Roth JH, Ross DC, King GJ. Endoscopic versus open carpal tunnel release: a randomized trial. *J Hand Surg Am.* 2003;28:475-480.
8. Braun RM, Rechnic M, Fowler E. Complications related to carpal tunnel release. *Hand Clin.* 2002;18:347-357.
9. Tung TH, Mackinnon SE. Secondary carpal tunnel surgery. *Plast Reconstr Surg.* 2001;107:1830-1843.

Relevant Review Articles

Cranford CS, Ho JY, Kalainov DM, Hartigan BJ. Carpal tunnel syndrome. *J Am Acad Orthop Surg.* 2007;15(9):537-548.

CHAPTER 3

GANGLION CYSTS

Gregory V. Sobol, MD

Ganglion cysts are the most common soft-tissue tumors of the hand and wrist. They occur more commonly in women than in men. Most frequently observed in patients between the second and fourth decades of life, they can be present at any age. Ganglions usually are isolated findings in particular locations, however, they have been reported to arise from multiple locations throughout the hand and wrist.

MECHANISM OF INJURY/ PATHOPHYSIOLOGY

Pathogenesis of ganglion cysts is unclear but several theories exist, including the following:

- **Herniation of synovial lining or benign tumors of synovial origin.** Dye studies have demonstrated communication between cysts and underlying joint; a one-way valve exists between the cyst and the joint. This theory is undermined by the lack of synovial lining within the cyst.[1]
- **Traumatic etiology** is supported by the demonstration of blood-tinged mucinous fluid in the cyst. The theory is that a rent is created in the underlying joint capsule or tendon sheath and that synovial fluid escapes and is walled off in the cyst. However, a specific antecedent traumatic event is recalled in only 10% of cases.

Rohde RS, Millett PJ, eds.
*Evaluation and Management
of Common Upper Extremity Disorders:
A Practical Handbook* (pp 35-48).
© 2011 Taylor & Francis Group.

- **The recurrent stress and microtrauma** theory is that overuse may stimulate mucin production by mesenchymal cells at the synovial-capsular interface.
- **Osteoarthritis** evident on radiographs often is associated with specific cysts of the hand and wrist.

KEY HISTORY POINTS

Patients with ganglion cysts usually seek evaluation due to cosmetic appearance, pain, alteration in size, and concerns about malignancy.

- The majority of patients with ganglion cysts have been aware of the cyst for some time.
- Most patients are pain-free, but pain sometimes is reported in association with activities or even at rest.
- The size of the cyst can fluctuate over days to months, often subsiding with rest and increasing with activity.
- Rarely is there an antecedent traumatic event.

KEY EXAMINATION POINTS

Location

- Certain locations are commonly associated with ganglion cysts and have a classic appearance on exam.
  - Dorsal wrist 60% to 70% (dorsal carpal ganglion cyst)
  - Volar radial wrist 13% to 20% (volar carpal ganglion cyst)
  - Dorsum of interphalangeal (IP) joints, distal more common than proximal (mucous cyst)
  - Volar surface of finger along tendon sheath 7% to 12% (retinacular cyst)

- Cysts have been reported at almost every joint in the hand and wrist. Less common areas include the following:
  - Radial hand and wrist (eg, basal joint, scaphotrapezotrapezoidal joint, first dorsal compartment, metacarpal bossing associated with cyst)
  - Extensor and flexor tendons of hand and wrist (eg, flexor carpi radialis tendon, extensor digitorum communis tendon, palmaris longus)
- **Nail changes** such as ridge formation can occur in the presence of mucous cysts at the distal interphalangeal (DIP) joint.
- **Palpation** of the mass may demonstrate it to be compressible but often very firm, sometimes firm enough that patients think it is bone. The mass is subcutaneous, often slightly mobile, and not adherent to underlying skin. Some are tender to palpation.
- Occult ganglion will demonstrate tenderness over the scapholunate ligament and pain with hyperextension of the wrist with normal radiographs and an otherwise normal examination.
- **Range of motion** usually is not affected but in some instances causes pain at the site. As always, underlying structures should be assessed for ligamentous injury or laxity or arthritic finding.
- **Neurologic impairment** secondary to ganglion cysts is rare but has been reported throughout the upper extremity. Nerves involved include the posterior interosseous, the ulnar nerve at the elbow and wrist, the median nerve at the wrist and its isolated motor branch, and the suprascapular nerve in the shoulder.
- **Allen's test** (Figure 3-1) is useful to assess radial and ulnar arterial flow when evaluating volar carpal ganglion cysts.
- **A transillumination test** can be performed by turning down the room lighting and shining light from

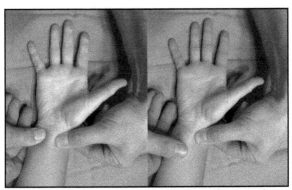

Figure 3-1. Allen's test. The patient makes a fist and releases digits several times to exsanguinate blood from the hand. The examiner compresses both the radial and ulnar arteries, preventing reperfusion of the hand. Release of the pressure on one of the arteries (in this case, the ulnar artery, right), allows reperfusion via that vessel. If the arch is complete, the entire hand will be reperfused by flow through that vessel. The procedure is repeated for the radial artery. *For the full-color version, see page CA-I of the Color Atlas.*

a penlight or small flashlight through the mass; light easily passes through this fluid-filled mass, differentiating it from a solid lesion.

Differential Diagnosis

- Extensive and varies for particular cyst and location
- Tenosynovitis
- Giant cell tumor
- Infection
- Accessory muscle
- Prominent bone (scaphoid, lunate, osteophyte, metacarpal base)
- Vascular lesion
- Other tumors (benign or malignant)

ADDITIONAL TESTING OR IMAGING

- **Radiographs** can be performed at the discretion of the physician. A radiograph of a ganglion cyst should not show any soft-tissue calcification, but might show soft-tissue shadows in the area. Arthritic changes—especially at the IP level, scaphotrapezotrapezoidal joint, and basal joint—might be noted. Occasionally, findings suggestive of ligamentous injury (scapholunate or lunotriquetral widening) can be identified.
- **Arthrograms** uncommonly are used and might show communication of the cyst with the underlying associated joint; notably, a **cystogram** will not show communication with the joint, consistent with the theory of one-way valves.
- **Magnetic resonance imaging** can be used in the case of a questionable differential diagnosis or if there is suspicion of an occult ganglion cyst. It can provide better anatomic detail as to location and complexity of the cyst.

TREATMENT OPTIONS: NONOPERATIVE

Reassuring the patient of the nonmalignant nature of the ganglion cyst generally is the most important nonoperative management.

Observation

- Most commonly recommended at initial evaluation with reassurance that this is benign and has about a 50% spontaneous resolution rate[2]
- Recommendation for follow-up if any change in size of cyst or nature of symptoms

Symptomatic Treatment

- Intermittent wrist splinting
- Nonsteroidal anti-inflammatory drugs
- Heat and/or ice
- Activity modification

Closed Rupture

- Some try to accomplish this technique, classically described as a "sharp blow with the Bible," using firm massage.
- This method is associated with high recurrence rates and risk of fracture (eg, metacarpal, wrist) with aggressive blow; it generally is not recommended.

Aspiration/Puncture

- Reported resolution rates are between 13% and 85% with aspiration or puncture.[3-5]
- The patient must be informed that complete pain resolution is unlikely, even if the cyst resolves, especially if there is underlying arthritis.
- Splinting and/or steroid injection following aspiration are performed commonly but have not been shown to provide benefit.
- Aspiration of a volar carpal ganglion cyst usually is not recommended due to proximity of neurovascular structures.
- Silk suture passed at right angles through the cyst, tied over the skin, and left in place for 3 weeks has been reported to have a 95% success rate, but fears of infection limit this method's popularity.

TREATMENT OPTIONS: OPERATIVE

Surgical excision can be performed for all cysts with different techniques depending on location. Bier block or

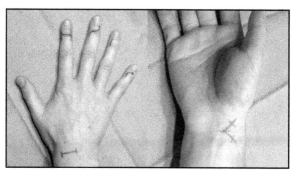

Figure 3-2. Many options are appropriate for excision of dorsal wrist lesions, mucous cysts, and volar ganglion cysts.

regional anesthetic with sedation generally is sufficient. Cysts can be removed through open incisions (Figure 3-2) and arthroscopically.

SURGICAL ANATOMY

Dorsal Carpal Ganglion Cysts

- Common structures encountered include the dorsal sensory branches of the radial and ulnar nerves, extensor tendons, wrist capsule, and the scapholunate ligament, which is the most common origin of the ganglion cyst.

Dorsal Carpal Ganglion Cysts: Arthroscopic

- Utilizes standard 3-4 and 6R wrist portals; the dorsal capsule and the scapholunate ligament are visualized.

Volar Carpal Ganglion Cysts

- Volar cysts most commonly are on the radial side of the wrist. Branches of the lateral antebrachial cutaneous nerve and superficial radial nerve should be protected. The flexor carpi radialis tendon and radial artery are visualized deeper in the wound. The cyst stalk generally emanates from the scaphotrapezial joint.
- Ulnar-sided cysts are associated with the flexor carpi ulnaris tendon and ulnar neurovascular bundle.

Volar Retinacular Cysts

- These are subcutaneous but superficial to the tendon proper and usually are located near the proximal digital flexion crease. They can be associated with the tendon sheath (A1 or A2 pulley). At risk are the digital neurovascular bundles.

Mucous Cysts

- Most commonly, mucous cysts are found at the DIP joint level. They can cause a rent in the extensor mechanism and pressure on the germinal matrix, deforming the nail plate. An underlying spur is often present.

PROCEDURES

Dorsal Carpal Ganglion Cyst: Open Excision

- The location of incision is marked prior to local anesthetic injection (if used).
- A forearm or upper arm tourniquet is used.

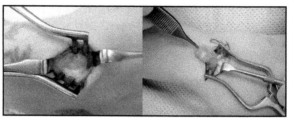

Figure 3-3. Excision of dorsal ganglion cyst. A transverse incision (left) generally yields a more cosmetic scar. The cyst is exposed between the second and fourth compartments and excised from its intercarpal origination (right). The cyst is full of translucent gelatinous fluid.

- Open excision utilizes a transverse incision along Langer's lines directly overlying the cyst (Figure 3-3).
- Sensory branches and extensor tendons are protected with right angle retractors.
- Dissection is continued between the second and fourth dorsal extensor compartments to the stalk of the cyst, which often emanates from capsular attachments at the scapholunate ligament.
- The stalk is excised with small portions of the surrounding capsule; the scapholunate ligament is preserved.
- The defect created in the dorsal capsule is not closed. The base of the stalk is often cauterized.

Dorsal Carpal Ganglion Cyst: Arthroscopic Excision

- Generally utilized only by those experienced and comfortable with wrist arthroscopy.
- A standard arthroscopic setup with the arthroscope in the 6R portal and a full radius shaver in the 3-4 portal is used.

- Shaving proceeds dorsally to the confluence of the dorsal capsule and the scapholunate ligament.
- The capsule and floor of the fourth dorsal compartment are removed.
- The cyst will be decompressed and a blush of ganglion fluid often is visible when the cyst wall is violated.
- Aggressive resection of the scapholunate ligament or extensor tendons should be avoided.

Volar Carpal Ganglion Cyst Excision

- Note: A preoperative Allen's test is useful to confirm ulnar arterial flow. If a documented ulnar artery occlusion exists, the risks must be weighed seriously and the surgeon and patient should be ready for possible vascular repair.
- Intravenous regional, regional block, or general anesthetic can be used.
- A longitudinal forearm incision and/or a chevron incision over the cyst, which often lies at the wrist flexion crease, is used. The wrist crease should not be crossed by a longitudinal incision.
- Superficial nerve branches are protected and the cyst is carefully dissected free from the radial artery; small branches will require cauterization.
- The flexor carpi radialis tendon is released and retracted ulnarly.
- If the cyst is significantly adherent to the radial vessels, a portion of the cyst wall can be left rather than jeopardizing the artery.
- The stalk of the cyst is identified and followed to the radiocarpal articulation.
- The stalk and a small portion of the associated capsule are excised; the defect in the capsule is not closed.

- The tourniquet is deflated prior to closure; perfusion is verified and hemostasis obtained. Failure to achieve hemostasis can lead to hematoma formation.
- Ulnar-sided volar cysts sometimes require release of Guyon's canal and possibly excision of the pisiform if arthritis is present.

Volar Retinacular Cyst Excision

- If needling the cyst fails or the cyst recurs and continues to be symptomatic, surgical excision is an option.
- Local anesthetic with a digital or forearm tourniquet usually is sufficient.
- An oblique incision is made over the cyst and the soft tissues are dissected bluntly to expose the cyst.
- The cyst is identified, the digital neurovascular bundles are protected, and the cyst is excised with a small portion of the adherent pulley.
- The incision is closed and a soft wrap is applied to allow early range of motion of the digit.

Mucous Cyst Excision

- This can be addressed under local anesthetic with a digital or forearm tourniquet.
- Multiple incisions have been described, including longitudinal, H-shaped, T-shaped, and curvilinear (see Figure 3-2).
- The cyst is identified and excised with the associated stalk from the DIP joint.
- The terminal tendon and germinal matrix are protected. The osteophytic spur from the distal phalanx is removed with a rongeur; this is key to preventing recurrence.[6]

- If primary closure cannot be completed, a rotational flap, skin graft, or healing by secondary intention are alternative options.
- A soft wrap is applied.

REHABILITATION

- Rehabilitation is minimal for most cysts. A period of soft-tissue rest to allow the wound to heal is followed by protected range of motion activities. Prolonged splinting can decrease recurrence slightly but also can increase stiffness.
- Therapy occasionally is necessary after wrist cyst excision but rarely needed after treatment of mucous and retinacular cysts.

OUTCOMES

Dorsal Carpal Ganglion Cysts

- Spontaneous resolution is as high as 50% and might be slightly higher in children.
- Closed rupture is successful in 22% to 66% but, because of the injury potential, is not recommended.
- Aspiration with or without steroid injections is reported to have a 10% to 40% resolution rate; success might increase with repeated aspirations.
- Surgical excision has recurrence rates of 4% if the associated capsule is excised compared to as high as 40% if just the cyst is excised.[2]

Volar Carpal Ganglion Cysts

- Aspiration is not recommended because of the proximity of neurovascular structures and a recurrence rate as high as 83%.
- Surgical excision of volar carpal ganglion cysts has a much higher recurrence than for dorsal: 33%.

Volar Retinacular Cysts

- Aspiration/rupture has a 50% to 70% success rate.
- There is a very low incidence of recurrence with excision.

Mucous Cysts

- Aspiration with or without steroid injection has a 50% recurrence rate.
- Surgical cyst excision and débridement of the DIP joint with osteophyte removal has a 2% recurrence rate; there is a much higher recurrence risk if only the cyst is excised.

POTENTIAL COMPLICATIONS

Similar complications exist for ganglion cysts of the hand and wrist but differ slightly by location.

- Aspiration/injection invokes risk to the surrounding neurovascular structures. Superficial sensory nerves, digital nerves, and even larger peripheral nerves can be at risk if attempts are made to aspirate volar ganglion cysts. Infection also is a risk with aspiration/injection and is more common with repeated attempts.
- Surgical excision risks include recurrence, infection, stiffness, instability, and neurovascular injury.

- Wrist stiffness is the most common adverse outcome. Avoiding prolonged immobilization postoperatively and leaving the capsular defect open are recommended to minimize stiffness.
- Aggressive capsular excision may compromise interosseous ligaments (most commonly the scapholunate ligament).
- The radial artery is intimately associated with volar radial ganglion cysts and is the most common vascular structure injured during the care of hand and wrist ganglion cysts.

REFERENCES

1. Psaila JV, Mansel RE. The surface ultrastructure of ganglia. *J Bone Joint Surg Br.* 1978;60:228-233.
2. Hooper G. Cystic swellings. In: Bogumill GP, Fleegler EJ, eds. *Tumors of the Hand and Upper Limb.* Vol 10. Edinburgh, Scotland: Churchill Livingstone; 1993:172-182.
3. Richman JA, Gelberman RH, Engber WD, Salamon PB, Bean DJ. Ganglions of the wrist and digits: results of treatment by aspiration and cyst wall puncture. *J Hand Surg Am.* 1987;12:1041-1043.
4. Korman J, Pearl R, Hentz VR. Efficacy of immobilization following aspiration of carpal and digital ganglions. *J Hand Surg Am.* 1992;17:1097-1099.
5. Zubowicz VN, Ishii CH. Management of ganglion cysts of the hand by simple aspiration. *J Hand Surg Am.* 1987;12:618-620.
6. Eaton RG, Dobranski AI, Littler JW. Marginal osteophyte excision in treatment of mucous cysts. *J Bone Joint Surg Am.* 1973;55:570-574.

Relevant Review Articles

Thornburg LE. Ganglions of the hand and wrist. *J Am Acad Orthop Surg.* 1999;7(4):231-238.

CHAPTER 4

DISTAL RADIUS FRACTURES

Rachel S. Rohde, MD and
Kimberly Mezera, MD

MECHANISM OF INJURY/ PATHOPHYSIOLOGY

The importance of the distal radius as the cornerstone of the wrist "joint" cannot be underestimated. Fractures of the distal radius have been noted as one of the most common injuries of the upper extremity, accounting for one-sixth of fractures seen in emergency departments.[1] These generally can be classified into groups that assist in planning management:

- **Low-energy** injuries often result from a fall from standing height onto an outstretched hand.
  - Often, an extension force results in dorsal displacement of the distal radius, usually in the metaphyseal area of the bone.
  - Minimal soft-tissue damage occurs.
  - Different fracture patterns result from asymmetrical loading (often including rotational force) through the hand. The mechanisms of injury have been associated with specific fracture patterns and have been used to define certain classification systems.[2]
- **High-energy** injuries include falls from heights, motorized accidents, and sports-related injuries.

49

Rohde RS, Millett PJ, eds.
Evaluation and Management
of Common Upper Extremity Disorders:
A Practical Handbook (pp 49-72).
© 2011 Taylor & Francis Group.

□ More complex fracture patterns and a higher incidence of associated soft-tissue injuries result.

□ The level of suspicion for associated injuries of the carpus, distal radioulnar joint (DRUJ), and ligamentous anatomy must be high.

- **Patient age** traditionally has been one factor used to guide management, however, with more widespread acceptance of new plating technology that diminishes the technical significance of bone quality on outcome and as patients remain active into later years, age is becoming a less important determinant of treatment.[3]

KEY HISTORY POINTS

- Age, hand dominance, occupation, and avocations of patient
- Mechanism of injury (particularly high/low energy)
- Timing of occurrence relative to seeking treatment
- Symptoms (pain, paresthesias)
- Associated injuries (eg, other fractures, head injury)

KEY EXAMINATION POINTS

Attention must be given to the obvious but fundamental basics, including appearance and function of skin, subcutaneous tissues, tendons, vessels, nerves, and bone.

- Skin should be inspected meticulously for any breech of integrity, regardless of how small. An open fracture historically has been an indication for emergent intervention; although the urgency currently is debated, open wounds certainly merit irrigation and débridement in the acute setting at minimum.

(TEXT CONTINUES ON PAGE 51)

COLOR ATLAS

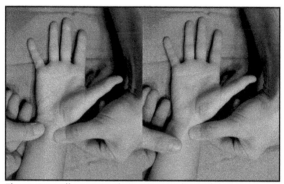

Figure 3-1. Allen's test. The patient makes a fist and releases digits several times to exsanguinate blood from the hand. The examiner compresses both the radial and ulnar arteries, preventing reperfusion of the hand. Release of the pressure on one of the arteries (in this case, the ulnar artery, right), allows reperfusion via that vessel. If the arch is complete, the entire hand will be reperfused by flow through that vessel. The procedure is repeated for the radial artery. *Also shown on page 38.*

- Vascular injury is uncommon, however, the index of suspicion for injury should be raised in the higher energy group.
- A complete neurological evaluation with special attention directed to the median nerve is essential.
  □ The **median nerve** often is directly in the zone of injury. An acute carpal tunnel syndrome may **evolve** because of edema or hematoma formation in the hours after a distal radius fracture and requires diligence in monitoring as well as prudent and timely carpal tunnel release in the acute setting.[4] Volar fragments or displacement can cause contusion of the median nerve, which often results in **immediate** post-injury symptoms that do not progress (and often resolve following closed reduction and immobilization).
  □ The ulnar nerve is not as often involved but must be assessed carefully in the setting of high-energy open fractures or severely displaced fractures.
- Tendons can become lacerated, interposed, or impaled on fracture fragments, especially in the widely displaced fracture patterns, and function of all flexor and extensor tendons must be assessed carefully.

ADDITIONAL TESTING OR IMAGING

- **Radiographs** are critical to evaluate the fracture pattern and offer much of the necessary information upon which treatment may be planned. There are 6 important radiographic parameters to consider when reviewing radiographs of a distal radius fracture (Figure 4-1).
  □ **Radial inclination:** Measured on the antero-posterior (AP) radiograph as the angle formed

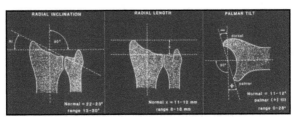

Figure 4-1. Three of the 6 radiographic parameters to be restored are radial inclination, radial length, and palmar (or volar) tilt. (Reprinted with permission from Weiland AJ, Rohde RS. *Acute Management of Hand Injuries.* Thorofare, NJ: SLACK Incorporated; 2009.)

by a line perpendicular to the longitudinal axis of the radius and a line from the tip of the radial styloid process to the ulnar corner of the radial articular surface. The average radial inclination is 22 to 23 degrees.

☐ **Palmar inclination** (often referred to as volar tilt): Measured on the lateral radiograph as the angle formed by a line perpendicular to the longitudinal axis of the radius and a line from the distal aspect of the dorsal and volar cortical rims. The average palmar inclination is 10 to 12 degrees.

☐ **Radial length**: Measured on the AP radiograph as the vertical distance between a line drawn at the tip of the radial styloid and a second line drawn at the articular surface of the ulnar head (both lines are oriented perpendicular to the long axis of the radius). The average radial length is 11 to 12 mm.

☐ **Articular congruity**: Measured on both AP and lateral radiographs. Ideally, 1 mm or less of displacement is optimal.

☐ **Ulnar variance**: Measured on the AP radiograph as the vertical distance between a line drawn parallel to the articular surface of the ulnar head and a second line parallel to the articular surface of the lunate facet. Neutral variance is the most common. Radiographs of the contralateral wrist may be used for comparison if needed, as patients' "normal" negative or positive ulnar variances vary.

- □ **Radial shift:** Measured on the AP radiograph as the distance between a line drawn at the most lateral tip of the radial styloid process and a line through the longitudinal axis at the center of the radial shaft.

- □ An additional radiographic view that can help one evaluate the palmar tilt and articular surface is obtained by orienting the X-ray tube 15 degrees in the proximal direction to the longitudinal axis or by raising the wrist approximately 30 degrees with the tube at neutral.

- □ Of special note is the **ulnar styloid fracture**. There is not widespread agreement regarding the treatment of these fractures; this continues to be a subject of controversy. The presence of an ulnar styloid fracture may be an important cue to look carefully at the carpus for associated injuries to the carpal bones and their ligamentous attachments; if examination reveals DRUJ instability following fixation of the distal radius fracture, consideration should be given to ulnar styloid fixation.

- **Computed tomography** can be used to define more accurately complex articular injuries including impaction injuries and DRUJ injury. It also can be used to identify occult carpal fractures and define the extent of the metaphyseal comminution associated with a particular fracture pattern.

- The usefulness of **magnetic resonance imaging** in this setting is increasing as the technology continues to advance; although it generally is not helpful to evaluate distal radius fractures, it can help one evaluate for ligamentous injuries about the wrist.

Treatment Options: Nonoperative Versus Operative Management

There are numerous classification systems cited in the literature[1]; the complete discussion of these is beyond the scope of this chapter. Classification systems allow reproducible descriptive diagnosis of bone and soft-tissue involvement independent of examiner, have prognostic and outcome significance, and because of these attributes are useful for guiding management. Often a simple description of the fracture serves as a valuable tool to communicate the resultant injury and assist in planning treatment.

Primary treatment options include nonoperative and operative options. Decision making with regard to management is refined throughout training and subsequent experience, but predictive factors for displacement of distal radius fractures have been reported. According to Mackenney et al,[5] key predictive factors include:

- **Patient age**: Fractures in those older than 80 years demonstrated early instability 10 times more frequently than those in patients younger than 30 years.
- **Comminuted fractures** were unstable 6 times more often than those without comminution.
- **Fractures with initial dorsal tilt at presentation** (5 to 10 degrees) were 5 times more likely to be unstable than those that maintained volar tilt.
- **Fractures with initial positive ulnar variance at presentation** were twice as likely to be unstable as those with neutral or negative variance (ie, radial shortening).

These predict early and late instability, which result in malunion and carpal malalignment. Consideration should be given to these factors when deciding the course of management.

TREATMENT OPTIONS: NONOPERATIVE

Nonoperative management essentially is limited to immobilization following any necessary closed reduction.

Reduction of the displaced fracture is most appropriately performed at the time of presentation in the emergency department setting with adequate pain control or appropriate sedation. High-quality injury radiographs are critical to the decision-making process and are excellent predictors of expected fracture stability after reduction. Anesthetic can be introduced into the fracture hematoma under sterile conditions in the emergency department or office setting to provide additional pain control during the procedure. Many different forms of splinting and casting have been used but all should follow the basic rule of leaving the fingers (including metacarpophalangeal [MCP] joints) free for range of motion and edema control exercises. Initial immobilization choice should allow for swelling (sugar tong splinting or bivalved casting). The period of immobilization ranges from 6 to 8 weeks in most cases; long arm immobilization generally is recommended at least for the initial 2 weeks.

TREATMENT OPTIONS: OPERATIVE

Operative management of distal radius fractures can involve closed reduction and percutaneous pin fixation, external fixation, open reduction and internal fixation, or a combination of these methods. Recent advancements in technology have led to a shift in fracture care allowing expanded treatment options for many fracture types.

Once considered a mainstay for fractures with little comminution and 1 or 2 large fragments, **closed reduction and percutaneous pin fixation** is quickly becoming less popular than internal fixation.

- It is helpful for isolated radial styloid fracture with minimal displacement (Chauffeur's fracture) or a fracture dislocation of the radiocarpal joint with small avulsion type fracture of the radial styloid.

- In the setting of a compromised soft-tissue envelope or open fracture, there may also be indications for provisional pin fixation.
- Disadvantage: The risks of fracture displacement and pin irritation often preclude immediate range of motion of the wrist.

External fixation once was considered the gold standard for many types of fractures of the distal radius, but now is used less commonly.

- Indicated for stabilization of a compromised soft-tissue envelope or as an adjunct to counter shortening in the case of severe bone comminution.
- Useful in the trauma setting as a temporizing measure with plans for conversion to definitive fixation at a later date.

Open reduction and internal fixation rapidly is becoming the new gold standard in the treatment of many types of distal radius fractures. There presently are more than 30 implant designs available for distal radius fracture fixation.[6] This advancement in technology is due in part to the development of a locking plate design that provides stable anatomic fixation secure enough to allow most patients immediate active range of motion; outcomes are described later in this chapter.

SURGICAL ANATOMY

The overall contours of the distal radius should be kept in mind when planning treatment; the volar surface is flat with a gentle slope while the dorsal side is convex, with the extensor pollicis longus (EPL) curving around Lister's tubercle. The 6 extensor compartments are associated intimately with the dorsal cortex of the radius, and approach to the bone is directed between compartments. The articular surface slants to the ulnar and volar side and consists of 2 concave facets that articulate with the scaphoid and lunate. Understanding the complex anatomy of the distal radius is integral to its reconstruction.

Because of the increased popularity of volar plating, the volar approach to the radius rapidly is becoming the most commonly used. However, the dorsal approach remains useful in many situations, and a surgeon treating distal radius fractures should be familiar with multiple approaches to allow for an intraoperative change of plans. A combined approach utilizing both may be indicated in complex intra-articular fracture patterns, carpal injuries, and in the reconstruction of malunions.

Volar Approach

The surgical anatomy of the volar approach includes the most distal part of the Henry approach to the forearm.

- An incision is made over the easily palpable flexor carpi radialis (FCR) tendon, located just ulnar to the radial artery.
- The sheath of the FCR may be opened and the tendon retracted to the ulnar side. Alternatively, the FCR sheath may be mobilized ulnarly intact with the interval developed at the radial border of the sheath.
- The floor of the FCR tendon sheath is incised longitudinally. The FCR tendon is retracted ulnarly and the radial artery retracted radially.
- The flexor pollicis longus tendon is mobilized ulnarly with a sweeping motion, exposing the pronator quadratus (PQ).
- The PQ is incised on the radial side and elevated to bring the distal radius into view. This approach affords limited access to the articular surface of the distal radius without compromising the important volar radiocarpal ligaments that keep the carpus from translating ulnarly and volarly.

- The brachioradialis (BR) acts as a deforming force and can prevent reduction of the radial styloid; release (tenotomy) of the BR allows improved fragment reduction.
- If direct access to the joint is necessary, it may be helpful to consider a dorsal approach or augmentation of the approach using arthroscopy.
- Direct exposure of an isolated lunate facet fragment can be accomplished volarly using a longitudinal incision parallel to the palmaris longus tendon and incising through the PQ.

Dorsal Approach

The dorsal approach is accomplished through straight longitudinal incisions and can be shifted radially or ulnarly, depending on the area of visualization needed.

- The incision is made longitudinally between the second and third dorsal compartments or the third and fourth compartments. Most commonly, the interval between the third and fourth compartments is developed. The EPL is mobilized from its sheath and retracted radially.
- The fourth compartment is maintained in its sheath and elevated subperiosteally in the ulnar direction.
- If necessary, the second dorsal compartment can be elevated to provide extensile access to the radius.
- An arthrotomy is made either longitudinally or in line with the fibers of the extrinsic wrist ligaments. This allows direct access to the articular surface of the radius for inspection or repair.
- After repair, the arthrotomy is closed and the extensor compartments replaced over the hardware.

- The EPL most commonly is placed back into its position but can be left outside the retinaculum to avoid ischemic injury.

Radial Approach

An alternative approach using a more radial interval between the first and second dorsal extensor compartments may help expose the radial styloid.

- The incision is made overlying the interval between the first and second dorsal compartments.
- The extensor retinaculum is incised and the compartment components retracted to allow access to the radial styloid.
- Care must be taken to protect the dorsal radial sensory nerve branch and the dorsal radial artery.

PROCEDURES

The choice of surgical procedure depends greatly on fracture configuration, accompanying soft-tissue injuries, patient factors, and surgeon experience. The following are brief guidelines and hints regarding performing the more common procedures.

Most injuries are addressed with the patient positioned in a supine position with the operative extremity on a radiolucent hand table. Regional anesthesia or general anesthesia can be used during the procedure. A tourniquet is applied to the operative upper arm, and the upper extremity is prepared and draped sterilely prior to starting the procedure. Attempted closed reduction and fluoroscopic visualization sometimes influences the choice of procedure immediately preoperatively and can be performed prior to exsanguination and tourniquet use. Prior to incision, the limb is exsanguinated and the tourniquet inflated per surgeon preference.

Open Reduction and Internal Fixation Using Volar Locking Plate

- The volar approach as described previously is utilized, allowing exposure of the distal radius. The fracture fragments and shaft proximal to the area are visualized.
- Plate designs differ according to number and direction of screws, available widths and lengths, and materials. A plate is chosen according to fracture characteristics, patient characteristics, and surgeon preference. Familiarity with the options and with use of each chosen plate is critical.
- Reduction generally is achieved using both direct and fluoroscopic visualization. Reduction goals are:
    □ Re-establishment of articular congruity by addressing the lunate facet and styloid fragments as well as other intra-articular fragments
    □ Restoration of appropriate radial inclination, radial height, and volar tilt
- Kirschner wires can be used for provisional fixation until definitive stability is achieved.
- The appropriate volar plate is chosen and placed as a buttress on the volar cortex of the distal radius. The plate should be long enough to allow stable proximal fixation and wide enough to enable capturing of fragments without interfering with the DRUJ.
- Distal locking screws are directed to be subchondral and thereby support the articular surface. Keep in mind that the concavity of the lunate facet demands that screws in this region be somewhat more proximal than more lateral screws to avoid intra-articular penetration (Figure 4-2).

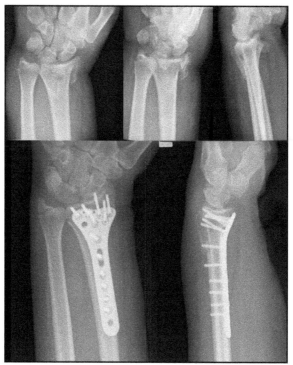

Figure 4-2. Preoperative (top) and postoperative (bottom) radiographs of a distal radius fracture addressed using a volar approach and a variable-angle volar locking plate. Preoperative radiographs show intra-articular extension, comminution, loss of radial height and inclination, and dorsal tilt. Postoperative radiographs demonstrate restoration of radiographic parameters and alignment of the ulnar styloid fragment. Note the subchondral location of the distal locking screws and that the length of these is just short of the dorsal cortex of the radius, preventing extensor tendon irritation. A longer than standard plate was used to obtain sufficient fixation proximal to the dorsal metaphyseal fracture.

- Confirmation of extra-articular subchondral screw placement should be made using the angulated lateral radiographic/fluoroscopic view described previously.
- Because of the stability provided by the locking mechanism, screws are unicortical. Penetration through the dorsal cortex can jeopardize tendons dorsally. Dorsal comminution and even normal dorsal anatomy can result in inadvertent prominence of screw tips; when measuring to determine screw length, one should err on the side of the shorter implant to avoid postoperative tendon irritation and rupture.
- Diaphyseal screws are bicortical and are inserted in standard fashion.
- Reduction, hardware placement, and hardware lengths are verified using multiple fluoroscopic views prior to closure.
- The wound is irrigated. The PQ can be repaired if preferred by the surgeon. The subcutaneous and skin layers are closed with the surgeon's preferred suture.
- Stability of the DRUJ and motion are evaluated and are addressed if necessary.
- Sterile dressings and a well-padded volar splint are applied.
- Timing of splint removal and hand therapy initiation depends upon patient motivation, compliance, and pain control as well as the stability of the fixed fracture.

Open Reduction and Internal Fixation Using Dorsal Plate

- The dorsal approach (Figure 4-3) described above is utilized to expose the distal radius. The articular surface is visualized.

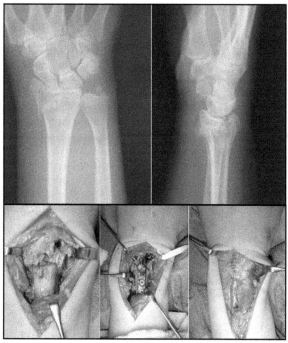

Figure 4-3. Anteroposterior and lateral radiographs demonstrate distal radius fracture with significant dorsal comminution (top). The dorsal approach allows visualization and fixation of fracture fragments using this buttress plate over which the soft tissues are closed (bottom). If desired, the extensor pollicis longus tendon can be transposed dorsal to the extensor retinaculum. (Reprinted with permission of Andrew Weiland, MD.)

- Manual distraction can allow assessment and reduction of fracture fragments. If necessary, a distractor can be utilized to assist with this. Impacted fracture fragment reduction can be achieved and maintained using provisional Kirschner wires. These should be inserted from a more distal direction to avoid obstruction of plate application.

- Many dorsal plate systems are available, and the appropriate selection is made based on requirements for fixation, patient anatomy, and surgeon preference. If necessary, the plate is contoured and/or sized appropriately. Ensure that the plate is as low profile as possible and that there are no sharp edges dorsally that might irritate the extensor tendons.
- The plate is secured to bone using multiple screws.
- Fracture reduction is evaluated throughout the procedure grossly and fluoroscopically. Stable fixation, restoration of the articular surface, and re-establishment of the radiographic parameters are the goals.
- The wound is irrigated and the extensor retinaculum closed; the EPL tendon often is left dorsal to the retinaculum. The skin is closed (with or without drain placement) per surgeon preference.
- Stability of the DRUJ and motion are examined.
- Sterile dressings and a volar plaster splint are applied. Following stable fixation of the fracture, rehabilitation is initiated when patient comfort and ability allow.

Open Reduction and Internal Fixation Using Radial Plate

Use of the direct approach allows fixation of the radial styloid. Remember that scapholunate or other intercarpal ligament injuries are common with isolated radial styloid fractures and that these are not addressed adequately using a limited radial approach. Radial plates and "nails" are available; the following is a brief guide to fixation using a radial plate.

- The direct lateral approach as described above is utilized.
- Manual reduction of the fracture is achieved; an elevator can be used if necessary to disimpact fragments.

- Provisional fixation is accomplished using Kirschner wire and the reduction evaluated fluoroscopically.
- The plate is contoured (if necessary) and applied to the lateral border of the radius to buttress the fracture.
- As with use of the volar plates, distal locking screws should be unicortical to avoid articular penetration (in this case, of the DRUJ). Proximal screws in the diaphyseal fragment can be bicortical.
- The reduction, hardware placement, and hardware lengths are evaluated fluoroscopically.
- The first dorsal compartment tendons are returned to their anatomic position. The wound is irrigated and the skin closed per surgeon preference.
- The wound is dressed with sterile dressings and a volar thumb spica splint is applied.
- Rehabilitation timing depends on patient comfort, compliance, and stability of fracture fixation.

External Fixation

Many external fixators are available for treatment of distal radius fractures. Some of these span the radiocarpal joint, using pins in the radial shaft and the index metacarpal; use of this type of external fixation is described. Nonspanning or nonbridging external fixators require the use of distal pins in the fracture fragments rather than in the metacarpal; application of these is beyond the scope of this text.

- A longitudinal incision is made along the radial border of the radial shaft approximately 5 cm proximal to the fracture site. The soft tissue is dissected carefully toward the interval between the BR and extensor carpi radialis longus. Branches of the lateral antebrachial cutaneous nerve are identified and protected.
- The interval between the BR and extensor carpi radialis longus is entered and the superficial branch

of the radial nerve is identified along the border of the BR; this nerve is in danger with percutaneous external fixator pin placement and is a primary reason to obtain adequate exposure.

- Positioning and insertion of the pins depends upon the chosen external fixator; some systems are accompanied by guides that determine placement of the pins relative to each other. If the chosen system does not include guides, 2.5- or 3-mm self-drilling pins can be placed approximately 3 cm apart on the radial shaft. Both pins should be bicortical; fluoroscopic guidance can be used to ensure appropriate penetration of the second cortex. Predrilling may be necessary to avoid fracture.
- A distal incision is made over the dorsoradial aspect of the index metacarpal. Again, exposure allows identification and protection of the superficial branch of the radial nerve.
- Two 2.5-mm pins are inserted into the index metacarpal. If a guide accompanies the system, this will determine the placement of these pins. Pin placement should be confirmed fluoroscopically.
- The incisions are irrigated and closed with nylon sutures.
- Bars are attached approximately 2 cm from the skin to the proximal and distal pairs of pins, and bar-bar connectors are used to attach these to each other to allow maintenance of the reduction. Some systems have built-in adjustment options that do not necessitate manipulation of these connectors. Fracture reduction is accomplished and the connectors are tightened to maintain the position.
- Ensure fluoroscopically that midcarpal and radiocarpal distraction are not excessive.
- Because this external fixator functions as an immobilizer, it is not necessary to apply a splint; soft dressings around the incisions and pin sites are sufficient.

Internal-External Fixation: Dorsal Distraction Plating

An alternative to external fixation for treating severely comminuted distal radius fractures has been described relatively recently.[7] Distraction plating utilizes a 3.5-mm plate to bridge the radiocarpal joint; a dorsal approach is utilized and fixation is achieved in the third metacarpal and the radial diaphysis. The articular surface can be reduced under direct visualization and fixed using Kirschner wires or screws; bone graft or bone graft substitutes also can be used when needed. Hardware must be removed following bone healing, at which time range of motion exercises can begin.

REHABILITATION

- A period of no weight bearing should be instituted until bone healing is confirmed. Premature resumption of activities can result in hardware failure and/or displacement of the fracture and consequent need for further intervention.
- Early active range of motion is encouraged when possible. Early motion of the digits is critical to prevent postoperative stiffness.
- Hand therapy for scar or wound management, edema control, tendon gliding, range of motion exercises, and eventual strengthening is beneficial.

OUTCOMES

Outcome following treatment of distal radius fractures is a topic of extensive ongoing research. Special emphasis is placed on functional outcome as well as potential complications.

Volar Plating

Most authors report good to excellent functional outcomes following volar plate fixation but also indicate the potential for a variety of complications. A multicenter prospective study of 150 patients managed using locking plates demonstrated good to excellent outcomes; noted complications included tendon inflammation (9) or rupture (2), loss of reduction (2), and screw loosening (2).[6] Similarly, 41 patients with distal radius fractures treated using volar locking plates demonstrated good to excellent functional outcomes. Complications included loss of reduction (4), tendon irritation (3), wound dehiscence (1), and MCP joint stiffness (1).[8] A group of 49 consecutive patients treated using volar locking plates were followed for 1 year postoperatively; excellent functional and radiographic results were achieved.[9] Although this last group did not report any complications, most authors describe various (usually minor) complications; patients should be made aware of the potential risks and surgeons should be diligent in identifying and addressing these issues.

Closed Reduction and Percutaneous Pin Fixation

Although closed reduction and percutaneous pin fixation has become less frequent as the use of internal fixation has increased, a retrospective review of 54 patients with 55 distal radius fractures treated with closed reduction and percutaneous pinning demonstrated excellent functional and radiographic outcomes at an average follow-up of almost 5 years with few complications.[10]

Internal Versus External Fixation Methods

Whether internal fixation methods lead to improved outcomes over external fixation methods is a subject of research. Evaluation of 46 patients randomized to be treated with a locked radial column plate (12), a locked volar plate (12), or augmented external fixation (22) was performed. The authors found that use of a locked volar plate led to improved outcomes in the first 3 months after fixation but that patients in all groups demonstrated similar excellent outcomes at 6 months and 1 year following fixation.[11] Similarly, a prospective study of 45 patients with distal radius fractures randomized to treatment using closed reduction and pin fixation or open reduction and internal fixation using a volar plate was performed. Although no significant functional differences existed by 1 year, better functional results were observed in the first several months following open reduction and internal fixation.[12] Studies such as these suggest that patients requiring quicker return to function for occupational or avocational activities may benefit from open reduction and internal fixation.

POTENTIAL COMPLICATIONS

Complications are associated both with the injury itself and with management; similarly, the incidence of certain complications varies depending on injury and treatment factors. Potential complications include:

- Infection
- Nerve or blood vessel injury (eg, median nerve paresthesias from retraction, superficial branch of radial nerve during pinning or external fixation)
- Scarring of the incision site and/or of tendons
- Digital or wrist stiffness

- Irritation from plate
- Tendon rupture
    - □ EPL tendon can rupture due to ischemia following nondisplaced distal radius fracture; patients should be warned to report any perceived dysfunction of the thumb.
    - □ Extensor tendon rupture has been reported with dorsal and volar plating techniques due to prominent hardware.
    - □ Flexor tendon rupture also has occurred after volar plating.
- Loss of fixation
- Unrecognized associated injuries
- Chronic regional pain syndrome

REFERENCES

1. Ilyas AM, Jupiter JB. Distal radius fractures—classification of treatment and indications for surgery. *Orthop Clin N Am.* 2007;38:167-173.
2. Fernandez DL. Fractures of the distal radius. Operative treatment. *Instr Course Lect.* 1993;42:73-88.
3. Chen NC, Jupiter JB. Current concepts review: management of distal radius fractures. *J Bone Joint Surg Am.* 2007;89:2051-2062.
4. Bauman TD, Gelberman RH, Mubarak SJ, Garfin SR. The acute carpal tunnel syndrome. *Clin Orthop Relat Res.* 1981;156:151-156.
5. Mackenney PJ, McQueen MM, Elton R. Prediction of instability in distal radius fractures. *J Bone Joint Surg Am.* 2006;88:1944-1951.
6. Jupiter JB, Marent-Huber M. LCP Study Group. Operative management of distal radial fractures with 2.4-millimeter locking plates: a multicenter prospective case series. Surgical technique. *J Bone Joint Surg Am.* 2010;92(Suppl 1 Pt 1):96-106.
7. Ginn TA, Ruch DS, Yang CC, Hanel DP. Use of a distraction plate for distal radial fractures with metaphyseal and diaphyseal comminution. Surgical technique. *J Bone Joint Surg Am.* 2006;88(Suppl 1 Pt 1):29-36.

8. Rozental TD, Blazar PE. Functional outcome and complications after volar plating for dorsally displaced, unstable fractures of the distal radius. *J Hand Surg Am.* 2006;31(3):359-365.

9. Osada D, Kamei S, Masuzaki K, Takai M, Kameda M, Tamai K. Prospective study of distal radius fractures treated with a volar locking plate system. *J Hand Surg Am.* 2008;33(5):691-700.

10. Glickel SZ, Catalano LW, Raia FJ, Barron OA, Grabow R, Chia B. Long-term outcomes of closed reduction and percutaneous pinning for the treatment of distal radius fractures. *J Hand Surg Am.* 2008;33(10):1700-1705.

11. Wei DH, Raizman NM, Botting CJ, Jobin CM, Strauch RJ, Rosenwasser MP. Unstable distal radial fractures treated with external fixation, a radial column plate, or a volar plate. A prospective randomized trial. *J Bone Joint Surg Am.* 2009;91(7):1568-1577.

12. Rozental TD, Blazar PE, Franko OI, Chacko AT, Earp BE, Day CS. Functional outcomes for unstable distal radial fractures treated with open reduction and internal fixation or closed reduction and percutaneous fixation. A prospective randomized trial. *J Bone Joint Surg Am.* 2009;91(8):1837-1846.

Relevant Review Articles

Chen NC, Jupiter JB. Current concepts review: management of distal radius fractures. *J Bone Joint Surg Am.* 2007;89:2051-2062.

Taras JS, Ladd AL, Kalainov DM, Ruch DS, Ring DC. New concepts in the treatment of distal radius fractures. *Inst Course Lect.* 2010;59:313-332.

CHAPTER 5

COMBINED RADIAL AND ULNAR FRACTURES

Robert R. L. Gray, MD and
Walter W. Virkus, MD

Combined radial and ulnar fractures, or both-bone forearm fractures, are common injuries to the upper extremity, especially in children. When evaluating these injuries and planning treatment, it must be understood that the radius and ulna are linked and form a ring. Forces seen by both bones are often translated through the entire ring, which includes the proximal radioulnar joint at the elbow and the distal radioulnar joint at the wrist. This fact necessitates that the adjacent joints in the setting of forearm fractures must be thoroughly evaluated throughout the treatment of these injuries.

MECHANISM OF INJURY/ PATHOPHYSIOLOGY

The vast majority of both-bone forearm fractures are the result of trauma. Traumatic mechanisms include:

- Fall on outstretched arm (most common)
- Direct crush injury
- Direct blow (very rare in both-bone and more common in single-bone forearm fractures and their variants)

Rohde RS, Millett PJ, eds.
Evaluation and Management
of Common Upper Extremity Disorders:
A Practical Handbook (pp 73-84).
© 2011 Taylor & Francis Group.

Though much less common, pathologic causes must be excluded:

- Malignancy
- Osteodystrophy

KEY HISTORY POINTS

- History of traumatic injury.
- Patient may notice swelling, ecchymosis, or deformity.
- Patient may complain of numbness, pain, or difficulty moving fingers.

KEY EXAMINATION POINTS

Diagnosis of the forearm fracture by history and examination is evident, usually even before radiographs are obtained. Associated injuries, however, can be subtle and must not be overlooked:

- Open fracture
- Compartment syndrome
- Radial head dislocation/fracture
- Distal radioulnar joint disruption
- Ipsilateral upper extremity fracture (eg, scaphoid, coronoid, distal humerus)
- Arterial injury (rare)

ADDITIONAL TESTING OR IMAGING

Radiographs and physical examination make the diagnosis. Computed tomography is only helpful in the instance of intra-articular extension, and even then rarely is needed to develop a treatment plan. Other additional testing, such as vascular studies or compartment pressure readings, is necessary only in the setting of concomitant vascular compromise or compartment syndrome.

TREATMENT OPTIONS

The intimate and specific anatomic relationship of the radius and ulna necessitates anatomic reduction of both-bone fractures. The anatomic bow of the radius must be maintained to allow full pronation and supination and unhindered elbow and wrist mechanics. Mild deviations can be accepted in pediatric fractures, especially if the fracture is more distal. Although conventionally thought to be unacceptable, rotational deformity of 30 degrees or more is required before the rotation of the forearm is hindered.[1] Typically, achieving this degree of rotational deformity without malalignment in another plane is unlikely.

TREATMENT OPTIONS: NONOPERATIVE

Nonoperative treatment in adults is reserved for fractures that essentially are nondisplaced. In children younger than 8 to 10 years of age, up to a centimeter of shortening may be accepted as long as the radial bow is maintained overall.[2]

TREATMENT OPTIONS: OPERATIVE

Operative treatment in children can be accomplished with open reduction and plate fixation, however, much success has been enjoyed with intramedullary fixation (eg, flexible titanium nails, Nancy nails, and Ender's rods). Often, only the ulna needs fixation, after which the radius reduces and the arm can be casted. It is important to be mindful of the increased incidence of compartment syndrome with nailing of both-bone forearm fractures.

In adults, open reduction and internal fixation with compression plating are the standard. Locking plates are reserved for fractures in osteoporotic bone or when the fracture line is too near the end of the bone to achieve 6 cortices of fixation on either side of the fracture line. A lag screw should be utilized if the fracture obliquity allows. We prefer using mini-fragment screws to lag across fracture lines of butterfly fragments and a compression plate to span the fractures.

Bone grafting usually is not necessary except in cases of significant bone loss. Often, cancellous autograft from the metaphyseal radius or olecranon can be used, or off-the-shelf demineralized bone matrix putty with cancellous allograft can fill voids, provided there is at least 20% cortical contact of the fracture ends. Typically, bone grafting is indicated only in revisions of nonunions.[3]

SURGICAL ANATOMY

Two separate incisions always should be used to address combined radial and ulnar fractures. Single-incision techniques have an unacceptably high rate of synostosis of the 2 bones (nearly 40%), compared with 2-incision approaches (less than 5%). Care should be taken to not disturb the interosseous membrane or to let bone graft or fragments settle along it. It is believed that these technical factors contribute to synostosis formation, especially in the proximal forearm.

Ulna

The incision is subcutaneous along its length. Care is taken to dissect between the flexor and extensor carpi ulnaris. The compression plate should be precontoured and placed on either the volar or dorsal cortex of the ulna so it is less subcutaneous and prominent. We typically use a dorsally applied plate.

Radius

The radius may be approached volarly (Figure 5-1), using the Henry approach, or dorsally, using the Thompson

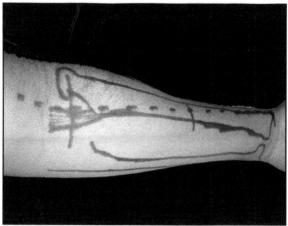

Figure 5-1. Anterior Henry approach to the radius. The incision (marked with a dashed line) extends from just lateral to the distal biceps tendon to the anterior aspect of the radial styloid. Often only a portion of the incision is needed for a simple, nonsegmental fracture.

approach. In the middle third, a direct radial approach may be employed (Figure 5-2), but this exposure is not extensile and should be avoided if there is any potential need to extend the exposure. Our preference is to treat radius fractures through an anterior approach; it is extensile and does not require direct dissection of the posterior interosseous nerve.

Anterior Approach

A line from the biceps tendon to the volar aspect of the radial styloid is drawn. The incision is along this line, and its placement and length are dictated by the fracture. Subcutaneous flaps are raised, and the muscle belly of the brachioradialis is encountered. This belly extends across the midline and proximally accounts for nearly 70% of the superficial layer. The pronator teres is found medially. The plane proximally is between

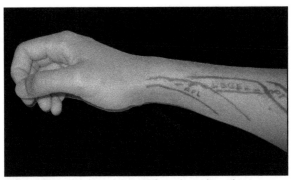

Figure 5-2. Direct lateral approach to the radius. This is a non-extensile approach that is suited for mid- to distal-third radial shaft fractures. Even with swelling from fracture hematoma, the bare area of the radius is palpable. Some release of the pronator teres insertion may be needed to access the bone for proximal plate placement.

these muscles. Care is taken to identify and protect the dorsal radial sensory nerve, which runs underneath the brachioradialis muscle. In distal exposures, the brachioradialis tendon (which is also the floor of the first extensor compartment) is released to aid in exposure of the intra-articular fracture fragments.

Proximally, the supinator muscle must be released to expose the bone. This is done carefully, and with the arm in full supination, to protect the posterior interosseous nerve, which pierces it and typically runs just a few millimeters from the insertion on the radius.

In the middle of the radius, the pronator teres insertion often needs to be partially, if not fully, released to expose the fracture and place the compression plate. While some authors prefer to step-cut the insertion and lengthen it, we will leave it completely released to scar back in place.

The distal radius has the flexor pollicis longus and the pronator quadratus origin and insertion, respectively.

Authors vary as to whether or not to repair the pronator quadratus insertion after plate fixation. Although some feel that a repaired pronator quadratus may lead to a single-muscle compartment syndrome that results in fibrosis, stiffness, and loss of supination, this has not been our experience and we routinely repair it if possible.

Posterior Approach

A line is drawn from the lateral epicondyle to the radial styloid with the arm in pronation. An incision is made along this line, its length and location dictated by the fracture.

Proximally, the interval between the extensor digitorum communis and the extensor carpi radialis brevis is entered. Beneath these, the supinator is encountered. It is important to carry out this dissection with the arm in pronation to protect the posterior interosseous nerve. If the surgeon desires to explore the nerve, the supinator may be divided in its midsubstance.

In the midportion of the radius is a bare area. This is bounded by the distal edge of supinator proximally and the pronator teres insertion distally.

The approach may be carried distally to the level of the abductor pollicis longus as it courses obliquely over the bone. It does not lend itself well to fixation of very distal radius fractures.

PROCEDURES

Closed reduction and intramedullary fixation is beyond the scope of this chapter, as it is employed primarily in pediatric fractures. Often, only the ulna is fixed with a flexible nail. Using flexible nailing in both-bone forearm fractures has been associated with increased risk of compartment syndrome.

External fixation usually is reserved for grossly contaminated open fractures with severe soft-tissue injury, or in staged treatment of infection, after extensive bony débridement. The primary goal with external fixation is restoration of length. It is much more difficult to restore radial bow and nearly impossible to compress using an external fixator. Therefore, these are primarily used in a salvage procedure as a temporizing measure. Care must be taken to dissect bluntly to the bone at the pin sites, especially in the radius, to avoid nerve or tendon injury. Small external fixation systems have been designed for the upper extremity. Pins should be spread to provide relative stability. Depending on the fracture location, fixator pins may be placed in the second metacarpal to span the radiocarpal joint.

Open reduction and internal fixation: Before beginning, it is useful to obtain radiographic views of the contralateral uninjured forearm to aid in restoring the appropriate radial bow and ulnar variance. Although most individuals have neutral to negative ulnar variance, it is useful to know if a patient is one of the few with positive variance before reduction commences.

- The patient is placed supine on an operating room table with hand table extension. Unless nerve exploration needs to be performed, we will often use a regional block.
- A nonsterile tourniquet is applied and the arm is prepared and draped and exsanguinated gently with an Esmarch bandage. The tourniquet is raised to 250 mm Hg.
- Typically, the easier fracture is approached first. This is almost always the ulna. Reducing and plating the ulna restores length and makes reduction of the radius easier. Care should be taken to ensure the ulna is out to length. Otherwise, anatomic reduction of the radius will be impossible.
- It is not unreasonable to provisionally fix the ulna and return to it once the radius is completely reduced and plated.

- Using one of the surgical approaches outlined above, the fracture is exposed.
- Using a small periosteal elevator, 1 to 2 cm of periosteum at the fracture edges is reflected, allowing visualization of the fracture keys.
- Using a bone-holding clamp, or "lobster claw," on each fragment, the ends are reduced. These may be provisionally fixed with a Kirschner wire or by clamping across a more oblique fracture. The fragments may also be provisionally reduced by clamping them to a compression plate, which is often necessary given the transverse nature of these fractures.
- The alignment is checked under fluoroscopy. Attention should be paid to the radial bow and the distal and proximal radioulnar joints. When using a straight compression or locking plate, the radial bow necessitates that the plate will be slightly eccentric on the bone proximally and distally. If there is no eccentric coverage of the plate, adequate bow has not been restored.
- In cases of butterfly fragments, we generally use mini-fragment screws to lag them to a larger fracture fragment, creating 2 main fracture fragments. Usually, these then are reduced readily and can be compressed using a standard compression plate.
- If the area of comminution or bone loss is too great, a locking plate in a bridged fashion can be used.
- Some manufacturers have developed fracture-specific plates that match the radial bow or contour of the ulna more precisely. These are seldom needed and are of the greatest utility when a mid-shaft fracture is combined with a distal fracture, especially in the radius.
- Bone grafting is only indicated when there is segmental bone loss. Graft is harvested from the olecranon or iliac crest depending on the size of

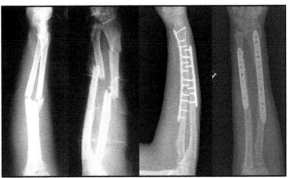

Figure 5-3. Pre- and postoperative radiographs of a both-bone forearm fracture; note the restoration of radial bow.

the defect, or off-the-shelf allograft demineralized bone matrix may be used.

- Recombinant bone morphogenic protein does not have clear indications in these fractures, and its use should be entertained in only the most challenging cases of revision surgery. Care must be taken in using it to avoid heterotopic bone formation as well as synostosis.
- Whichever plate is used, a minimum of 6 cortices of purchase in each fragment is optimal. Standard AO techniques should be employed, including pre-bending of the plate to prevent gapping on the far cortex, as well as eccentric drilling and sequential tightening of the screws to provide compression.
- If used, locked plates should be utilized with the manufacturer's drill guides to ensure threading of the screws into the plate. Beware of contouring these plates, as the locking mechanism may be affected by plate bending.
- Pre- and postoperative radiographs demonstrating this technique are shown in Figure 5-3.

REHABILITATION

The arm is immobilized in a short arm volar and dorsal plaster splint after plate fixation. After intramedullary rodding or nonoperative management, patients initially are placed in a long arm cast and then mobilized after 1 week in a short arm cast. No weight bearing is allowed through the limb for a period of 6 weeks. This is increased gradually depending on the stability of the fixation.

Early range of motion of the hand and elbow is of paramount importance. The hand is elevated to help prevent swelling and stiffness of the digits. A sling is issued for comfort, but the patient is encouraged to come out of it several times per day for range of motion exercises.

Physical or occupational therapy with putty for strengthening and range of motion stretching is initiated gently at 6 weeks. By 12 weeks, aggressive therapy for range of motion and strengthening is initiated.

OUTCOMES

Results after open reduction and compression plating of both-bone forearm fractures are typically excellent.[4] Union is achieved in excess of 95% of cases. Patients with appropriate reduction and fixation usually can be expected to return to full activity without difficulty, although recent research suggests a potential for persistent weakness compared to the contralateral side.

Results are complicated primarily by symptomatic hardware (usually of the ulna), and malreduction, which can result in proximal or distal radioulnar joint pain and disability. Much less common are nonunions, infections, and neurovascular injury.[5]

POTENTIAL COMPLICATIONS

- Malunion
- Nonunion
- Synostosis (much higher incidence with 1-incision approaches)
- Neurovascular injury (posterior interosseous nerve injury in proximal dorsal exposure, radial sensory nerve, and radial artery in anterior approach)
- Complex regional pain syndrome
- Infection (especially in open fractures)
- Symptomatic hardware (especially on the ulna if it is not positioned volarly)

REFERENCES

1. Dumont CE, Thalmann R, Macy JC. The effect of rotational malunion of the radius and the ulna on supination and pronation. *J Bone Joint Surg Br*. 2002;84:1070-1074.
2. Bae DS. Pediatric distal radius and forearm fractures. *J Hand Surg*. 2008;33:1911-1923.
3. Moghaddam A, Elleser C, Biglari B, Wentzensen A, Zimmerman G. Clinical application of BMP 7 in long bone non-unions. *Arch Ortho Trauma Surg*. 2010;130(1):71-76.
4. Droll K, Perna P, Potter J, Harniman E, Schemitsch E, McKee M. Outcomes following plate fixation of fractures of both bones of the forearm in adults. *J Bone Joint Surg Am*. 2007;89:2619-2624.
5. Stern P, Drury W. Complications of plate fixation of forearm fractures. *Clin Orthop Relat Res*. 1983;175:25-29.

Relevant Review Articles

Moss JP, Bynum DK. Diaphyseal fractures of the radius and ulna in adults. *Hand Clin*. 2007;23(2):143-151.

CHAPTER 6

LATERAL EPICONDYLITIS

*David C. Gerhardt, MD and
Jennifer Moriatis Wolf, MD*

Lateral epicondylitis, or "tennis elbow," is a common cause of lateral elbow pain in adults, affecting between 1% and 3% of the population each year.[1,2] It is a multifactorial pathologic condition predominantly involving the origin of the extensor carpi radialis brevis (ECRB) and often is associated with repetitive wrist extension.[3]

MECHANISM OF INJURY/ PATHOPHYSIOLOGY

The specific pathophysiology of lateral epicondylitis has not yet been fully described, but it is believed to be a failed reparative process rather than active inflammation. Overuse injuries leading to microtearing of the ECRB and occasionally the extensor digitorum communis (EDC) have been proposed as the initiating step in the degenerative cascade.[4] The resultant microscopic pathologic change at the common extensor origin has been termed *angiofibroblastic tendinosis* and includes the following characteristics[5,6]:

- Lack of inflammatory cells
- Vascular proliferation with nonfunctional vascular buds
- Immature fibroblast infiltration

Rohde RS, Millett PJ, eds.
*Evaluation and Management
of Common Upper Extremity Disorders:
A Practical Handbook* (pp 85-100).
© 2011 Taylor & Francis Group.

- Mucopolysaccharide infiltration
- Disorganized, hypercellular adjacent tissue

The common extensor origin may be vulnerable to injury due to anatomic hypovascular zones: one zone at the lateral epicondyle and the other zone 2 to 3 cm distal to the extensor origin.[7] These areas are potential watershed zones predisposing the ECRB to injury and impaired healing potential. Imbalance in the autonomic regulation of vasoconstriction and vasodilation also can contribute to or exacerbate a failed reparative process at the common extensor origin.[8,9]

KEY HISTORY POINTS

- Lateral elbow pain, usually poorly defined by the patient (may radiate down forearm)
- Possible history of repetitive activity
- Often no specific inciting event or injury (usually insidious onset)
- Pain is exacerbated by activities requiring active wrist extension or passive wrist flexion with the elbow extended (may complain of weakened grip and difficulty lifting objects)[10,11]
- Morning stiffness after periods of decreased elbow activity
- Dull ache that sometimes lasts through the day
- Pain with lifting when the forearm is in neutral

KEY EXAMINATION POINTS

- Maximal tenderness slightly anterior and distal to the lateral epicondyle (over the origin of the ECRB and EDC).[11]
- Pain elicited with resisted wrist extension and digit extension.[11]

- Occasionally may have tenderness over the apex of the lateral epicondyle proper.
- Positive Thompson's test: The patient's shoulder is flexed to 60 degrees, the elbow is extended, the forearm is pronated, and the wrist is extended to 30 degrees. Pain is reproduced when the examiner applies pressure to the second and third metacarpals to stress the ECRB.[12]
- Positive chair test: Pain is reproduced when the patient lifts a light chair by the chair back with the elbow extended and the forearm pronated.[12]
- Grip strength can be tested and may be weak compared to that of the contralateral side.

ADDITIONAL TESTING OR IMAGING

Lateral epicondylitis is primarily a clinical diagnosis, and imaging is generally not needed for diagnosis. However, imaging can provide useful information for preoperative planning, defining the extent of the disease, and ruling out other sources of elbow pain.

- **Radiographs** are helpful to assess for fractures, dislocations, radio-opaque loose bodies, or degenerative joint disease. In general, they are low yield in lateral epicondylitis; no specific findings are associated with lateral epicondylitis. However, calcifications or exostosis of the epicondyle near the extensor origin occasionally are seen.[3,5]
- **Ultrasound** may show calcification of the common extensor tendon, focal hypoechoic regions within the tendon, complete or partial discrete cleavage tears, and diffuse heterogeneity.[13,14] Sensitivity varies between 64% and 82% and is highly operator dependent.[15]
- **Magnetic resonance imaging** (MRI) shows increased T1 signal within the extensor tendon as well as tendon thickening in 90% to 100% of symptomatic

elbows.[16-18] MRI is useful in quantifying the degree of tendon involvement as well as ruling out other intra-articular pathology but should be reserved for recalcitrant symptoms, as signal change in the extensor origin may be a common finding in patients older than 40 years.[17]

TREATMENT OPTIONS: NONOPERATIVE

The mainstay of treatment for lateral epicondylitis is nonoperative management.

Observation combined with rest and activity modification may lead to improvement in symptoms. A wait-and-see approach has been supported in the literature with an 83% success rate at 1-year follow-up.[19,20]

Oral nonsteroidal anti-inflammatory drugs (NSAIDs) commonly have been used to treat acute lateral epicondylitis, and although the disease is characterized as a noninflammatory condition, NSAIDs may relieve symptoms from associated synovitis and inflammation in the surrounding soft tissues.[6,11] Given the associated gastrointestinal side effects, lack of short-term functional improvements, and lack of long-term treatment differences, oral NSAIDs have a limited role.

Splints commonly include proximal forearm bands or cock-up wrist splints. They may inhibit the maximal contraction of the extensors and flexors leading to decreased tension of the common extensor origin and allowing time to heal.[21] There are no definitive data showing the superiority of either forearm bands or cock-up splints, but forearm bands are routinely prescribed to increase functional use of the affected arm.[22-24] Long-term efficacy of these devices has not been proven.[25]

Physical and/or occupational therapy has been used widely and may include manipulation, deep friction massage, strengthening and stretching protocols, and instruction regarding activity modification.[10] Stretching protocols of the extensor origin include bringing the wrist into flexion with the elbow extended and the forearm pronated.[22] Eccentric strengthening therapy may induce hypertrophy of the musculotendinous unit and reduce strain. It has demonstrated a positive effect without causing more disability but has not shown benefit over stretching alone or stretching combined with concentric strengthening.[26,27]

Steroid injections have been shown to be effective in treating the acute pain of lateral epicondylitis. Short-term results (follow-up to 6 weeks) have shown significant pain relief.[19,28,29] However, longer term (12 weeks to 12 months) follow-up has shown no difference when compared to NSAID or placebo.[11,19,28] When compared to the injection of lidocaine alone, outcomes at 1 year did not differ.[30]

- Risks associated with steroid injections include skin depigmentation, fat atrophy, decreased collagen production, and impaired tenocyte replication.[11,31]

Botulinum toxin injections may temporarily partially paralyze the extensors, allowing for healing in a less tensioned environment. Although some studies conflict regarding efficacy outcomes at 3 months, a recent multicenter, randomized, controlled trial showed a clear benefit with pain relief and improved function at 4 months with botulinum toxin as compared to placebo injection.[32-34] Detrimental weakness in patients who performed intricate work with their hands has been reported.[33,34]

Autologous blood injections have been used in the treatment of refractory lateral epicondylitis and are hypothesized to induce a healing cascade through increased levels of transforming growth factor-β and basic fibroblast growth factor.[35] Success rates of 50% with 1 injection and 79% with an additional 1 or 2 injections have been reported.[35]

- Injection is performed using 2 cc autologous blood drawn from an antecubital vein mixed with 1 cc of lidocaine (Figure 6-1).

Other injections including alcohol, carbolic acid, glucosaminoglycans, and more recently, the use of platelet-

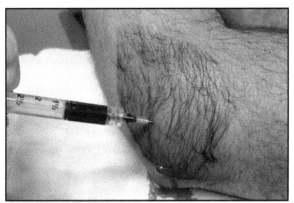

Figure 6-1. Autologous blood is injected into the extensor carpi radialis brevis origin.

rich plasma have been tried, but they are less widely used and are not as well supported in the literature.[10]

Extracorporeal shock wave therapy has been evaluated in meta-analysis studies and has not shown any notable effect.[36]

Other therapeutic interventions including **laser therapy, topical medications,** and **acupuncture** have been evaluated and have shown mixed results in small series, without compelling evidence to support their routine use.

TREATMENT OPTIONS: OPERATIVE

Surgical treatment in lateral epicondylitis is reserved for cases refractory to nonoperative interventions for 6 months to 1 year. It has been estimated that the general community orthopedic surgeon would have about a 5% rate of operative intervention.[37] Many different surgical techniques have been described, including releasing the common extensor origin (open or percutaneously, with or without repair), débriding the pathologic ECRB tissues, releasing the posterior interosseous nerve, arthroscopic release, anconeus rotation, and lateral epicondyle denervation.

SURGICAL ANATOMY

- The lateral epicondyle has been described as a pyramid-shaped prominence.[38] The anconeus originates from the posterior aspect; the ECRB and EDC origins lie on the anterior face. The extensor carpi radialis longus (ECRL) and brachioradialis origins are more cephalad along the anterior aspect of the supracondylar ridge.[11]
- The ECRL is muscular at is origin and visibly contrasts the tendinous ECRB.[11]
- The common extensor origin is a combination of the ECRB and EDC origins, there is often poor definition between the borders of these to tendons.[39]
- The pathology of lateral epicondylitis occurs in the more superior and slightly deeper fibers of the ECRB.[11]
- The lateral collateral ligament complex originates from the apex of the epicondyle and includes the ulnar collateral ligament, radial collateral ligament, and the annular ligament.[11]
- The posterior interosseous nerve enters the supinator just distal to the radial head and enters the radial tunnel.

PROCEDURES

The open procedure, as described by Nirschl, allows for release or lengthening of the ECRB, with or without débridement of the extensor origin, and is the most common surgical approach for lateral epicondylitis.[5] Percutaneous release of the extensor origin has been described and is done using a No. 11 blade under local lidocaine infiltration.[40] Arthroscopic approaches have been used for treatment of lateral epicondylitis and have shown equivalent outcomes to open procedures.[41]

Lateral Epicondylar Open Débridement

- The patient is positioned supine with the operative extremity resting on a hand table. An upper arm tourniquet is used; the prepared site should allow access to the distal portion of the humerus.
- An incision is marked 3 to 4 cm in length from 2 cm proximal and just anterior to the lateral epicondyle to a point 1 cm distal to the level of the joint.
- The limb is exsanguinated and the tourniquet is inflated.
- The skin is incised and the soft tissues are dissected to expose the longitudinal border of the ECRL and extensor aponeurosis.
- The border between the ECRL and the EDC is divided longitudinally in line with the fibers (Figure 6-2). The ECRL and EDC are retracted anteromedially to expose the ECRB. The ECRL can be sharply dissected off the anterior ridge to allow for additional visualization of the extensor origin if necessary.
- Degenerative tissue appears gray, shiny, abnormal or necrotic, with consistent fibrous granulation tissue at the ECRB origin. This tissue should be excised as part of the débridement procedure.
- If present, lateral epicondylar exostoses may be removed with a rongeur or rasp. Stimulating bleeding at this site may serve to induce further healing, and limited decortication of the lateral epicondyle by osteotome, rongeur, or drilling has been described.[42,43]
- Care should be taken not to create instability at the elbow by releasing the lateral collateral ligaments off of the posterior lateral epicondyle.
- After the wound is irrigated, the split in the fascia can be repaired with absorbable sutures prior to closure with sutures of choice.

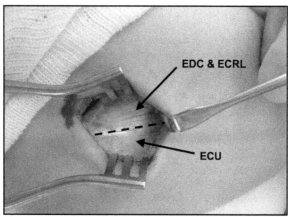

Figure 6-2. Surgical exposure. The extensor carpi radialis longus (ECRL)/extensor digitorum communis (EDC) and the extensor carpi ulnaris (ECU) are divided to expose the underlying extensor carpi radialis brevis (ECRB).

- The wound is dressed with sterile dressings. A 10-day period of immobilization in a splint is preferred by some surgeons.

REHABILITATION

- After a period of immobilization (immediate to 10 days postoperatively), range of motion exercises are started.[44,45]
- Patients may benefit from wearing a wrist support splint for 10 to 14 days followed by gradual return to activities.[11]
- Strengthening exercises are started after 6 weeks.
- Sports such as tennis or golf may be commenced after 8 to 10 weeks.[11]

OUTCOMES

Time and nonoperative treatments for lateral epicondylitis usually result in good outcomes. Corticosteroid use may be most beneficial during the period of acute onset of symptoms. No single nonsurgical treatment has demonstrated definitive superiority. For recalcitrant, chronic lateral epicondylitis, surgical options provide a good success rate.

- **Nonoperative treatments** including corticosteroid injection, physical therapy, or observation have shown success rates of 69%, 91%, and 83%, respectively, at 1 year.[19] The vast majority of cases respond to conservative therapy but may take up to 18 months to attain full recovery.
- **Open treatment** with débridement for chronic lateral epicondylitis has shown a 97% improvement over the patient's preoperative status, with an 85% return-to-work rate with complete relief of pain at 3 months.[5] Additional studies show an 83% to 94% relief of pain with ECRB release and débridement.[46,47]
- **Arthroscopic treatment** has shown high success rates (93% to 100% were "better" or "much better") and early return to work, averaging 15 days.[41,44,48,49] However, only 62% to 80% of patients were reported to have complete pain relief at 2 years.[41,49]
- **Open versus arthroscopic** treatments have not shown significantly different results at 6 months, but arthroscopic treatment groups may return to work earlier.[44,50]

POTENTIAL COMPLICATIONS

- Skin depigmentation and fat atrophy following corticosteroid injections

- Persistent pain from posterior interosseous nerve entrapment initially not recognized[51]
- Neuroma of the posterior cutaneous nerve of the forearm with open surgery[52]
- Heterotopic ossification following arthroscopy[53]
- Posterolateral rotary instability following overly aggressive débridement with injury to the lateral ulnar collateral ligament, in both arthroscopic and open surgeries[54]
- Infection
- Recurrence

REFERENCES

1. Verhaar JA. Tennis elbow. Anatomical, epidemiological and therapeutic aspects. *Int Orthop.* 1994;18(5):263-267.
2. Allander E. Prevalence, incidence, and remission rates of some common rheumatic diseases or syndromes. *Scand J Rheumatol.* 1974;3(3):145-153.
3. Goldie I. Epicondylitis lateralis humeri (epicondylalgia or tennis elbow). A pathogenetical study. *Acta Chir Scand Suppl.* 1964;57(Suppl 339):331.
4. Nirschl RP. Prevention and treatment of elbow and shoulder injuries in the tennis player. *Clin Sports Med.* 1988;7(2):289-308.
5. Nirschl RP, Pettrone FA. Tennis elbow. The surgical treatment of lateral epicondylitis. *J Bone Joint Surg Am.* 1979;61(6A):832-839.
6. Nirschl RP, Ashman ES. Elbow tendinopathy: tennis elbow. *Clin Sports Med.* 2003;22(4):813-836.
7. Bales CP, Placzek JD, Malone KJ, Vaupel Z, Arnoczky SP. Microvascular supply of the lateral epicondyle and common extensor origin. *J Shoulder Elbow Surg.* 2007;16(4):497-501.
8. Ljung BO, Forsgren S, Friden J. Substance P and calcitonin gene-related peptide expression at the extensor carpi radialis brevis muscle origin: implications for the etiology of tennis elbow. *J Orthop Res.* 1999;17(4):554-559.
9. Smith RW, Papadopolous E, Mani R, Cawley MI. Abnormal microvascular responses in a lateral epicondylitis. *Br J Rheumatol.* 1994;33(12):1166-1168.

10. Faro F, Wolf JM. Lateral epicondylitis: review and current concepts. *J Hand Surg Am.* 2007;32(8):1271-1279.

11. Calfee RP, Patel A, DaSilva MF, Akelman E. Management of lateral epicondylitis: current concepts. *J Am Acad Orthop Surg.* 2008;16(1):19-29.

12. Scher DL, Wolf JM, Owens BD. Lateral epicondylitis. *Orthopedics.* 2009;32(4).

13. Levin D, Nazarian LN, Miller TT, et al. Lateral epicondylitis of the elbow: US findings. *Radiology.* 2005;237(1):230-234.

14. Connell D, Burke F, Coombes P, et al. Sonographic examination of lateral epicondylitis. *AJR Am J Roentgenol.* 2001;176(3):777-782.

15. Miller TT, Shapiro MA, Schultz E, Kalish PE. Comparison of sonography and MRI for diagnosing epicondylitis. *J Clin Ultrasound.* 2002;30(4):193-202.

16. Mackay D, Rangan A, Hide G, Hughes T, Latimer J. The objective diagnosis of early tennis elbow by magnetic resonance imaging. *Occup Med (Lond).* 2003;53(5):309-312.

17. Potter HG, Hannafin JA, Morwessel RM, et al. Lateral epicondylitis: correlation of MR imaging, surgical, and histopathologic findings. *Radiology.* 1995;196(1):43-46.

18. Steinborn M, Heuck A, Jessel C, Bonel H, Reiser M. Magnetic resonance imaging of lateral epicondylitis of the elbow with a 0.2-T dedicated system. *Eur Radiol.* 1999;9(7):1376-1380.

19. Smidt N, van der Windt DA, Assendelft WJ, et al. Corticosteroid injections, physiotherapy, or a wait-and-see policy for lateral epicondylitis: a randomised controlled trial. *Lancet.* 2002;359(9307):657-662.

20. Szabo RM. Steroid injection for lateral epicondylitis. *J Hand Surg Am.* 2009;34(2):326-330.

21. Froimson AI. Treatment of tennis elbow with forearm support band. *J Bone Joint Surg Am.* 1971;53(1):183-184.

22. Nirschl RP. Tennis elbow. *Orthop Clin North Am.* 1973;4(3):787-800.

23. Van De Streek MD, Van Der Schans CP, De Greef MH, Postema K. The effect of a forearm/hand splint compared with an elbow band as a treatment for lateral epicondylitis. *Prosthet Orthot Int.* 2004;28(2):183-189.

24. Struijs PA, Smidt N, Arola H, et al. Orthotic devices for the treatment of tennis elbow. *Cochrane Database Syst Rev.* 2002(1):CD001821.

25. Struijs PA, Kerkhoffs GM, Assendelft WJ, Van Dijk CN. Conservative treatment of lateral epicondylitis: brace versus physical therapy or a combination of both—a randomized clinical trial. *Am J Sports Med.* 2004;32(2):462-469.

26. Martinez-Silvestrini JA, Newcomer KL, Gay RE, et al. Chronic lateral epicondylitis: comparative effectiveness of a home exercise program including stretching alone versus stretching supplemented with eccentric or concentric strengthening. *J Hand Ther.* 2005;18(4):411-420.

27. Svernlov B, Adolfsson L. Non-operative treatment regime including eccentric training for lateral humeral epicondylalgia. *Scand J Med Sci Sports.* 2001;11(6):328-334.

28. Hay EM, Paterson SM, Lewis M, Hosie G, Croft P. Pragmatic randomised controlled trial of local corticosteroid injection and naproxen for treatment of lateral epicondylitis of elbow in primary care. *BMJ.* 1999;319(7215):964-968.

29. Lewis M, Hay EM, Paterson SM, Croft P. Local steroid injections for tennis elbow: does the pain get worse before it gets better? Results from a randomized controlled trial. *Clin J Pain.* 2005;21(4):330-334.

30. Altay T, Gunal I, Ozturk H. Local injection treatment for lateral epicondylitis. *Clin Orthop Relat Res.* 2002;398: 127-130.

31. Wong MW, Tang YY, Lee SK, et al. Effect of dexamethasone on cultured human tenocytes and its reversibility by platelet-derived growth factor. *J Bone Joint Surg Am.* 2003;85-A(10):1914-1920.

32. Placzek R, Drescher W, Deuretzbacher G, Hempfing A, Meiss AL. Treatment of chronic radial epicondylitis with botulinum toxin A. A double-blind, placebo-controlled, randomized multicenter study. *J Bone Joint Surg Am.* 2007;89(2):255-260.

33. Hayton MJ, Santini AJ, Hughes PJ, et al. Botulinum toxin injection in the treatment of tennis elbow. A double-blind, randomized, controlled, pilot study. *J Bone Joint Surg Am.* 2005;87(3):503-507.

34. Wong SM, Hui AC, Tong PY, et al. Treatment of lateral epicondylitis with botulinum toxin: a randomized, double-blind, placebo-controlled trial. *Ann Intern Med.* 2005;143(11):793-797.

35. Edwards SG, Calandruccio JH. Autologous blood injections for refractory lateral epicondylitis. *J Hand Surg Am.* 2003;28(2):272-278.

36. Buchbinder R, Green SE, Youd JM, et al. Shock wave therapy for lateral elbow pain. *Cochrane Database Syst Rev.* 2005;(4):CD003524.

37. Nirschl RP. Elbow tendinosis/tennis elbow. *Clin Sports Med.* 1992;11(4):851-870.

38. Boyer MI, Hastings H 2nd. Lateral tennis elbow: "Is there any science out there?" *J Shoulder Elbow Surg.* 1999;8(5):481-491.

39. Greenbaum B, Itamura J, Vangsness CT, Tibone J, Atkinson R. Extensor carpi radialis brevis. An anatomical analysis of its origin. *J Bone Joint Surg Br.* 1999;81(5):926-929.

40. Baumgard SH, Schwartz DR. Percutaneous release of the epicondylar muscles for humeral epicondylitis. *Am J Sports Med.* 1982;10(4):233-236.

41. Baker CL Jr, Murphy KP, Gottlob CA, Curd DT. Arthroscopic classification and treatment of lateral epicondylitis: two-year clinical results. *J Shoulder Elbow Surg.* 2000;9(6): 475-482.

42. Peters T, Baker CL Jr. Lateral epicondylitis. *Clin Sports Med.* 2001;20(3):549-563.

43. Das D, Maffulli N. Surgical management of tennis elbow. *J Sports Med Phys Fitness.* 2002;42(2):190-197.

44. Peart RE, Strickler SS, Schweitzer KM Jr. Lateral epicondylitis: a comparative study of open and arthroscopic lateral release. *Am J Orthop.* 2004;33(11):565-567.

45. Owens BD, Murphy KP, Kuklo TR. Arthroscopic release for lateral epicondylitis. *Arthroscopy.* 2001;17(6):582-587.

46. Organ SW, Nirschl RP, Kraushaar BS, Guidi EJ. Salvage surgery for lateral tennis elbow. *Am J Sports Med.* 1997;25(6):746-750.

47. Rosenberg N, Henderson I. Surgical treatment of resistant lateral epicondylitis. Follow-up study of 19 patients after excision, release and repair of proximal common extensor tendon origin. *Arch Orthop Trauma Surg.* 2002;122 (9-10):514-517.

48. Baker CL Jr, Baker CL 3rd. Long-term follow-up of arthroscopic treatment of lateral epicondylitis. *Am J Sports Med.* 2008;36(2):254-260.

49. Mullett H, Sprague M, Brown G, Hausman M. Arthroscopic treatment of lateral epicondylitis: clinical and cadaveric studies. *Clin Orthop Relat Res.* 2005;439:123-128.

50. Szabo SJ, Savoie FH 3rd, Field LD, Ramsey JR, Hosemann CD. Tendinosis of the extensor carpi radialis brevis: an evaluation of three methods of operative treatment. *J Shoulder Elbow Surg.* 2006;15(6):721-727.

51. Werner CO. Lateral elbow pain and posterior interosseous nerve entrapment. *Acta Orthop Scand Suppl.* 1979;174: 1-62.

52. Dellon AL, Kim J, Ducic I. Painful neuroma of the posterior cutaneous nerve of the forearm after surgery for lateral humeral epicondylitis. *J Hand Surg Am.* 2004;29(3): 387-390.

53. Sodha S, Nagda SH, Sennett BJ. Heterotopic ossification in a throwing athlete after elbow arthroscopy. *Arthroscopy.* 2006;22(7):801-803.

54. Kalainov DM, Cohen MS. Posterolateral rotatory instability of the elbow in association with lateral epicondylitis. A report of three cases. *J Bone Joint Surg Am.* 2005;87(5):1120-1125.

Relevant Review Articles

Calfee RP, Patel A, Dasilva MF, Akelman E. Management of lateral epicondylitis: current concepts. *J Am Acad Orthop Surg.* 2008;16(1):19-29.

CHAPTER 7 | CUBITAL TUNNEL SYNDROME

Michael Darowish, MD

MECHANISM OF INJURY/ PATHOPHYSIOLOGY

- Cubital tunnel syndrome is a clinical syndrome of pain and paresthesias in the distribution of the ulnar nerve caused by slowing of ulnar nerve conduction velocity as the nerve passes behind the medial epicondyle of the elbow.
- It is the second most common nerve compression syndrome of the upper extremity.
- Ulnar neuropathy, the underlying cause of cubital tunnel syndrome, likely is multifactorial.
- Altered transmission of nerve impulses results from focal ischemia caused by one or more of the following mechanisms:

Nerve Compression

There are several anatomic sites at which the ulnar nerve can be compressed (Figure 7-1):
- Arcade of Struthers
    - Fascial bands between the medial triceps and medial intermuscular septum
    - Uncommon site of compression, except if incompletely released during anterior transposition

Rohde RS, Millett PJ, eds.
*Evaluation and Management
of Common Upper Extremity Disorders:
A Practical Handbook* (pp 101-122).
© 2011 Taylor & Francis Group.

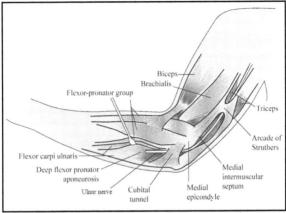

Figure 7-1. Nerve compression can occur at several anatomic regions in the medial upper arm, elbow, and forearm. (Adapted from Elhassan B, Steinmann SP. Entrapment neuropathy of the ulnar nerve. *J Am Acad Orthop Surg.* 2007;15:672-681.)

- Medial intermuscular septum
  - Generally not a site of compression for a native ulnar nerve unless the nerve subluxates anteriorly
  - Previously transposed ulnar nerve can be compressed by an incompletely released septum
- Flexor carpi ulnaris fascia
  - Superficial (eg, Osborne's ligament and arcuate ligament)
  - Deep-investing fascia
- Venous leash
- Space-occupying lesions (eg, ganglia, lipomata, synovial hypertrophy, bone spurs, loose bodies)
- Anconeus epitrochlearis (anomalous muscle connecting the olecranon and medial epicondyle found in 10% of patients undergoing cubital tunnel surgery)
- Cubitus valgus (tardy ulnar nerve palsy resulting from nerve traction from valgus elbow angulation, often due to old injury)

- Prolonged elbow flexion
    - Decreases volume of the cubital tunnel by up to 55% and increases pressure within the cubital tunnel 7-fold
    - A 20-fold increase in pressure within the cubital tunnel is demonstrated during elbow flexion and flexor carpi ulnaris contraction
- External compression (leaning on the elbow)

Traction

- Elbow flexion causes nerve excursion (and associated friction) and stretching of the nerve itself

KEY HISTORY POINTS

- Numbness or tingling in small and ring fingers
- Can be accompanied by discomfort, weakness, fatigability, difficulty opening jars/bottles, and loss of coordination
- Can awaken patient from sleep
- Includes dorsal hand numbness (can help distinguish from more distal compression at Guyon's canal, where dorsum of hand is spared; however, the dorsal cutaneous branch often is spared even in severe ulnar nerve compression at the elbow)
- Exacerbated by prolonged elbow flexion (typing, talking on phone, or sleeping with elbow flexed), leaning on elbow (driving)

KEY EXAMINATION POINTS

- Subjective loss of sensation in small finger and ulnar half of ring finger
- Weakness or absence of motor function
    - Abduction/adduction of fingers (interossei)
    - Crossing fingers (interossei)

- □ Flexor digitorum profundus to ring and small fingers
- Atrophy, most notable in the first web space due to denervation of the first dorsal interosseous muscle
- Elbow examination
  - □ Palpate ulnar nerve behind medial epicondyle; note irritability with pressure or anterior subluxation of the nerve with elbow flexion.
  - □ Assess carrying angle for presence of cubitus valgus.
  - □ Evaluate for swelling, which can be indicative of a space-occupying lesion.
- Special signs of differing extents of ulnar neuropathy
  - □ Froment's sign: Instead of using the first dorsal interosseous to adduct the thumb to hold paper between the thumb and index finger, the patient will compensate for loss of the interosseous muscle by flexing the interphalangeal joint of the thumb (median innervated) to pinch. This can be seen with severe ulnar neuropathy.
  - □ Wartenberg's sign: The small finger rests in an abducted position due to loss of interosseous musculature and intact abductor digiti minimi. This generally is seen in low ulnar nerve palsy.
  - □ Clawing: The ring and small fingers assume a resting position of metacarpophalangeal hyperextension and proximal and distal interphalangeal flexion due to loss of the intrinsics (lumbricals) with intact flexor digitorum superficialis and profundus. This is most notable in the ring and small fingers due to preservation of the median innervated lumbricals to the index and long fingers. Clawing is typically seen in low ulnar nerve palsy due to preservation of the proximally innervated flexor digitorum profundus to the ring and small fingers.

With more proximal ulnar nerve compression, the flexor digitorum profundus to the ring and small fingers are affected, and clawing is less noticeable, though still may be present.

- Provocative maneuvers
    - Tinel's sign: Percussion of the ulnar nerve at the posterior elbow elicits electric "shocks" in the small finger; this can be positive in 24% of asymptomatic individuals.[1]
    - Scratch collapse test: The patient resists bilateral external rotation of the shoulder. The skin overlying the ulnar nerve then is scratched with the examiner's fingernail. Bilateral shoulder external rotation then is retested immediately. A positive test demonstrates temporary loss of external rotation strength on the affected side.
    - Elbow flexion test: The elbow is held in full flexion for 60 seconds; a positive test reproduces paresthesias in the ring and small fingers. Asking the patient to extend the wrist as well can increase tension on the nerve; however, this maneuver also stretches the nerve at Guyon's canal, potentially confounding results. This can be positive in 10% of individuals without ulnar nerve compression.
    - Elbow flexion and compression test: The elbow is held in full flexion for 60 seconds while additional manual compression of the ulnar nerve at the cubital tunnel is performed. A positive test reproduces ulnar distribution paresthesias; this test reportedly exhibits 91% sensitivity.
    - Spurling's test: The patient's neck is extended and rotated toward the involved side; axial compression on the patient's head reproducing or worsening upper extremity symptoms is suggestive of foraminal nerve compression in the cervical spine.

□ Hoffmann's sign: The patient's hand is held loosely, and the tip of the long finger is flicked. Thumb interphalangeal joint or index finger proximal and/or distal interphalangeal joint reflexive contraction is considered a positive sign. While this can be found in approximately 10% of the general population, in the setting of arm numbness, this may be suggestive of myelopathy or upper motor neuron involvement.

Differential Diagnosis

- Cervical spine
    - □ C8 impingement
    - □ Syrinx
    - □ Tumor
- Peripheral neuropathy
    - □ Diabetes
    - □ Vitamin B12 deficiency
    - □ Alcoholism
    - □ Hypothyroidism
- Ulnar nerve compression at Guyon's canal
- Medial epicondylitis
- Thoracic outlet syndrome
- Apical lung tumor

ADDITIONAL TESTING OR IMAGING

- **Radiographs** are appropriate if there is a history of trauma to assess for valgus malunion, symptomatic hardware, impinging osteophytes, or heterotopic ossification.
- **Magnetic resonance imaging** is indicated only if a space-occupying lesion (such as a tumor) is suspected.

- **Nerve conduction study/electromyography** (EMG) is the most common diagnostic test used in cases of ulnar neuropathy.
  - □ This test can be used to confirm the diagnosis, document severity, evaluate for radiculopathy or peripheral neuropathy, and assess for other sites of compression, including thoracic outlet syndrome. It is not necessary to make the diagnosis, which is a clinical one.
  - □ The test should be performed with the elbow flexed at 70 to 90 degrees; flexing the elbow further may increase false-positive results.
  - □ Focal slowing of the motor conduction velocity by greater than 10 m/s across the elbow is diagnostic of ulnar neuropathy.
  - □ Axonal involvement can manifest on the EMG as positive sharp waves and fibrillation potentials in the abductor digiti minimi or first dorsal interosseous.
  - □ Many patients have symptoms but normal electrodiagnostic studies; this might be due to the dynamic, positional, intermittent nature of nerve compression at the elbow or to sampling error (if undiseased fascicles may be tested). By the time changes are detectable on EMG or nerve conduction study, the symptoms sometimes will be advanced. Favorable results have been reported by several authors in patients treated operatively with persistent symptoms despite negative electrodiagnostic studies.

TREATMENT OPTIONS: NONOPERATIVE

- Nonoperative treatment is indicated in mild cases with intermittent sensory impairment. It can be tried in patients with weakness, but with less expectation

for complete symptom resolution. We do not recommend that nonoperative treatment be considered for
patients with atrophy.

- Activity modification
  - □ Avoidance of elbow flexion beyond 45 degrees
    - • Patients who use keyboards consistently
      should be instructed to elevate the chair and
      lower the keyboard height in order to main-
      tain this limitation of flexed elbow posture.
  - □ Eliminating external pressure on postero-
    medial elbow
  - □ Avoid triceps-strengthening exercises
- Extension splinting
  - □ Splinting should be done at night to prevent
    elbow flexion while sleeping.
  - □ Elbow should be in slight flexion (35 to
    45 degrees).
  - □ Options include wrapping a towel or pillow
    around the elbow, wearing an elbow pad
    backward, or having a thermoplastic splint fab-
    ricated by a hand therapist to fit the patient.
- Anti-inflammatory medications

TREATMENT OPTIONS: OPERATIVE

- Indicated for patients with continued symptoms
  despite appropriate nonoperative management and
  patients with severe nerve compression (demonstrated by atrophy, altered 2-point discrimination,
  nerve conduction study or EMG).
- Choice of procedure depends upon patient factors
  (cause of neuropathy, comorbidities) and surgeon
  factors (experience, surgeon preference).
- General or regional anesthesia with sedation is
  used. If regional block is chosen, supplemental
  local anesthetic infiltration in the upper medial arm
  might be necessary.

SURGICAL ANATOMY

- The ulnar nerve originates as the terminal branch of the medial cord of the brachial plexus. It travels distally along the posterior border of the medial intermuscular septum and is covered by the fascia along the medial aspect of the triceps. Approximately 8 cm proximal to the epicondyle, a fascial band can be encountered connecting the medial head of the triceps to the medial intermuscular septum (the Arcade of Struthers), which can serve as a point of iatrogenic kinking during transposition.

- At the level of the elbow, the ulnar nerve passes posterior to the medial epicondyle and medial to the olecranon within a bony groove. Occasionally, muscle fibers can be seen extending from the medial border of the olecranon to the medial epicondyle, compressing the nerve (anconeus epitrochlearis).

- The ulnar nerve then passes through the cubital tunnel, entering the flexor carpi ulnaris between the ulnar and humeral heads of the muscle. The nerve lies within the flexor carpi ulnaris, deep to the muscle fibers and underneath an investing layer of deep fascia.

- Within the floor of the cubital tunnel, the fibers of the posterior band of the medial collateral ligament can be identified and are at risk of injury with aggressive deep dissection in this area.

- The ulnar nerve has no branches proximal to the elbow. It may give off articular sensory branches to the elbow joint; these are variable. Within the flexor carpi ulnaris, the ulnar nerve gives off motor branches to both heads of the flexor carpi ulnaris.

- The medial antebrachial cutaneous nerve runs anterior to the medial intermuscular septum. Distally, the medial antebrachial cutaneous nerve has a variable branching pattern, giving off 1 to 3 branches. These can be found proximal to, at, or distal to the epicondyle. These branches are located in the sub-cutaneous tissues just superficial to the fascia of the flexor carpi ulnaris. Because of their proximity, and because they cross over the surgical field, they are at risk for transection during cubital tunnel surgery and can be the source of painful neuroma formation should this occur. As such, careful dissection to iden-tify these nerves can prevent this complication.

PROCEDURES

In Situ Decompression: Open

- Indications for in situ decompression with-out transposition currently are controversial. Contraindications include anterior subluxation of the ulnar nerve with elbow flexion either pre- or postoperatively. Severe ulnar neuropathy is a rela-tive contraindication.
- Decompression can be performed open or endo-scopically; endoscopic cubital tunnel release is beyond the scope of this chapter.
- The patient is positioned supine with the af-fected extremity on a hand table unless additional procedures are planned that require alternative positioning.
- A tourniquet is applied to the upper arm; use of a sterile tourniquet following preparation and draping can allow for tourniquet removal if extension of the incision very proximally is needed intraoperatively.
- An incision is made along the course of the ulnar nerve originating at the level of the cubital tunnel and extending distally. Nerve compression proxi-mal to the cubital tunnel is extremely rare, but if proximal compression is suspected either by palpa-tion over the nerve proximally or by nerve conduc-tion study or EMG, the incision should be extended proximally to release the offending structures.

- The subcutaneous soft tissues are dissected carefully through fat down to the fascia of flexor carpi ulnaris. The branches of the medial antebrachial cutaneous nerve (which pass superficial to the flexor carpi ulnaris fascia within the subcutaneous layer) should be identified and protected.
- The ulnar nerve is identified passing posterior to the medial condyle in the cubital tunnel.
- The superficial fascia of the flexor carpi ulnaris is released. The muscle fibers are teased apart gently and the deep investing fascia of the flexor carpi ulnaris overlying the nerve is released. Care must be taken not to injure the motor branches to the flexor carpi ulnaris.
- The deep investing fascia must be released 10 cm distal to the midpoint of the retrocondylar groove, as bands can be encountered that far distally.[2]
- The nerve should not be released circumferentially, as this can destabilize the nerve within the cubital tunnel, allowing subluxation and thus necessitating transposition.
- The elbow should be taken through a full range of motion to confirm that the nerve does not subluxate over the medial epicondyle in flexion.
- If subluxation does not occur, the wound is closed in layers. A bulky soft dressing is applied.
- Elbow motion is allowed within days after surgery.

Anterior Subcutaneous Transposition

- There are several indications for anterior subcutaneous transposition:
  - □ Anterior subluxation of the nerve after simple decompression
  - □ Orthopedic implants preclude return of the nerve to its native position

□ No definitive compression is found during in situ release (can be suggestive of a traction phenomenon, which is not well addressed by in situ decompression)

□ Failed in situ decompression[3]

□ Cubitus valgus

□ Overhead-throwing athletes

□ Surgeon preference

■ Procedure

□ The patient is positioned and the ulnar nerve exposed similarly as with in situ decompression.

□ The incision should be extended proximally to allow mobilization of the nerve as far proximally as the intermuscular septum.

□ Circumferential neurolysis is completed to allow for free mobilization of the nerve; attempts are made to preserve vascularity of the nerve.

□ The medial intermuscular septum must be identified and excised to prevent compression of the nerve by the taut edge as the nerve is transposed anteriorly. Several large veins invariably run along the septum, and meticulous hemostasis should be maintained.

□ The ulnar nerve is gently placed anterior to the medial epicondyle.

□ A sling can be created to prevent subluxation of the nerve posteriorly into the cubital tunnel. Different slings can be created by using the following methods:

• A proximally based flap of the flexor pronator fascia can be sutured to the subcutaneous layer to keep the nerve anterior to the epicondyle.

• The deep subcutaneous tissue can be sutured to the flexor pronator fascia.

- A sling of intermuscular septum released proximally can be used as a turn-down flap onto the flexor pronator fascia.
□ The nerve should be inspected in its anterior position during full elbow range of motion to confirm that there is no evidence of kinking or compression.

Intramuscular (Transmuscular) Transposition

- Holds a theoretical advantage of placing the nerve into a well-vascularized bed, as well as providing a more direct line post-transposition, avoiding potential kinking as the nerve plunges deep into the fibers of the flexor carpi ulnaris. However, this requires more substantial dissection of the flexor pronator musculature and therefore a prolonged recovery.
- Ulnar nerve decompression and intermuscular septum resection are completed as described.
- Proximally and distally based flaps are created in the superficial fascia of the flexor pronator mass (Figures 7-2A and B).
- Deep longitudinal septae within the flexor pronator mass must be incised to create a soft bed for the nerve, preventing iatrogenic nerve compression (Figure 7-2C).
- A trough is formed within the muscle fibers in which the nerve will sit (Figure 7-2D).
- The nerve is placed into its anteriorly transposed position (Figure 7-2E).
- The superficial fascial flaps of the flexor pronator mass are repaired in a lengthened position with 2-0 absorbable suture. Care must be taken to avoid nerve compression with this repair; the surgeon should be able to place a finger underneath this flap (Figure 7-2F).

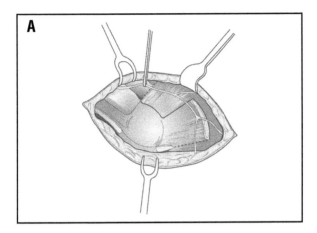

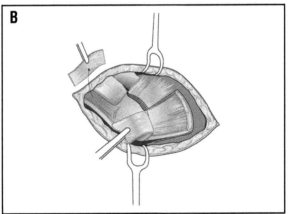

Figure 7-2. (A and B) Z-flaps are elevated from the flexor pronator mass, and a segment of the medial intermuscular septum is excised. (Adapted from Mackinnon SE, Novak CB. Compression neuropathies. In: Green DP, Hotchkiss RN, Pederson WC, Wolfe SW, eds. *Green's Operative Hand Surgery*. 5th ed. Edinburgh, Scotland: Elsevier Churchill Livingstone; 2005.)

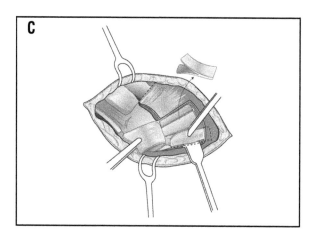

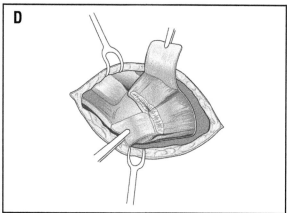

Figure 7-2. (C) Vertical fascial septa are incised within the flexor pronator muscle mass to provide a soft bed for the transposed nerve. (D) A trough is created within the flexor pronator muscle mass in which the nerve will sit. (Adapted from Mackinnon SE, Novak CB. Compression neuropathies. In: Green DP, Hotchkiss RN, Pederson WC, Wolfe SW, eds. *Green's Operative Hand Surgery*. 5th ed. Edinburgh, Scotland: Elsevier Churchill Livingstone; 2005.)

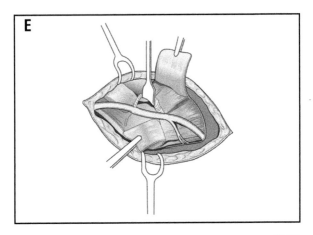

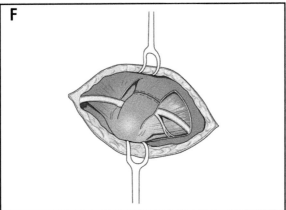

Figure 7-2. (E) The ulnar nerve is transposed into its anterior position within the flexor pronator mass. (F) The previously elevated fascial flaps are repaired in a z-lengthened position. (Adapted from Mackinnon SE, Novak CB. Compression neuropathies. In: Green DP, Hotchkiss RN, Pederson WC, Wolfe SW, eds. *Green's Operative Hand Surgery*. 5th ed. Edinburgh, Scotland: Elsevier Churchill Livingstone; 2005.)

- The nerve should be examined closely as it crosses the intermuscular septum and as it exits the flexor pronator musculature to confirm the absence of compression by fascial edges.
- The elbow should be taken through a range of motion to verify that no kinking of the nerve occurs.
- Postoperatively, active motion and nerve gliding can be initiated at 1 week. Formal strengthening should be delayed for 6 weeks, and unrestricted return to manual labor typically takes approximately 3 months.

Submuscular Transposition

- Ulnar nerve decompression and intermuscular septum resection are completed as described.
- The insertion of the flexor pronator mass is identified at the medial epicondyle and its fascia is incised 1 to 2 cm distal to the epicondyle.
- A periosteal elevator is used to elevate the muscle bluntly and reflect it distally.
- The median nerve is identified lying on the brachialis.
- The ulnar nerve is placed into a transposed position; the new position will be medial and parallel to the median nerve.
- The nerve should be examined as it crosses the intermuscular septal area and as it exits the flexor pronator musculature to confirm the absence of compression by fascial edges.
- The flexor pronator mass is repaired back to its insertion with nonabsorbable suture (Learmonth technique) or repaired with fascial lengthening as described in the intramuscular technique above (Dellon technique).
- Postoperatively, the elbow is maintained at 90 degrees for 1 week, at which time motion can be

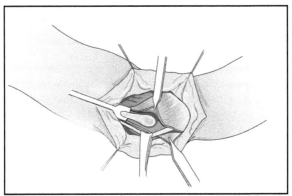

Figure 7-3. An osteotome is used to resect approximately 20% (5 mm) of the epicondyle. (Adapted from Hiethoff S, Millender LJ. Medial epicondylectomy. In: Gelberman RH, ed. *Operative Nerve Repair and Reconstruction*. Philadelphia, PA: Lippincott Williams and Wilkins. 1991;1087-1096.)

initiated. Formal strengthening should be delayed for 6 weeks, and unrestricted return to manual labor typically takes approximately 3 months.

Medial Epicondylectomy

- In situ decompression is performed as described.
- The medial epicondyle is exposed subperiosteally.
- An osteotome is used to resect a portion of the epicondyle and medial intermuscular septum. It is recommended that only 20% of the epicondyle (ie, 5 mm) be removed in order to preserve the entire insertion of the anterior band of the medial collateral ligament (Figure 7-3).
- The bone edges are smoothed with a rasp.
- The periosteal sleeve is repaired with the elbow in extension using inverted 3-0 absorbable suture.

- The elbow is taken through a range of motion to confirm nerve gliding and the absence of subluxation.
- Postoperatively, the patient is placed in a long arm splint; active motion is initiated at 10 days.

REHABILITATION

Postoperative rehabilitation depends on the procedure chosen, as described. Occupational therapy may be prescribed if needed for nerve gliding, desensitization, or ultimately, strengthening.

OUTCOMES

- A history of elbow trauma, presence of atrophy, advanced patient age, alcoholism, diabetes, or revision surgery portend poorer outcome.
- Patients with only sensory symptoms have a better prognosis for recovery. A 1989 meta-analysis reported nearly 100% excellent results, regardless of surgical technique employed, if symptoms were mild preoperatively. The same authors reported a 33% failure rate in patients with severe compression preoperatively, regardless of surgery performed.[4]
- Duration of symptoms correlates with poorer outcome.
- No single surgical technique has been definitively shown to be superior. Reports supporting each technique exist, but few comparative studies are available.
- Several studies have suggested that in situ decompression works well in patients with normal or only mildly abnormal nerve conduction study or EMG, but has inferior results in patients with moderate or severe compression.

- In situ decompression versus anterior transposition
  - □ Two recent meta-analyses have shown no significant difference in outcomes in patients following simple decompression or anterior transposition. One recommended decompression as a reasonable alternative to transposition because it is a simpler procedure; the other observed a (nonsignificant) trend toward improved outcomes with transposition.[5,6]
- Sub- or intramuscular transposition is not recommended for overhead-throwing athletes.

POTENTIAL COMPLICATIONS

- Incomplete relief of symptoms
  - □ Incomplete decompression (reported in up to 57% of cases with continued symptoms)
  - □ Iatrogenic compression following transposition
    - Incomplete release of flexor carpi ulnaris fascia distally
    - Incomplete release or excision of intermuscular septum proximally
    - Incomplete release of vertical septa within flexor pronator mass
    - Compression by repaired fascia following intra- or submuscular transposition
  - □ Second site of nerve compression (eg, cervical disc, Guyon's canal)
  - □ Irreversible nerve changes despite appropriate care
- Iatrogenic nerve subluxation
- Iatrogenic nerve injury
- Symptomatic neuroma formation from injured medial antebrachial cutaneous nerve branches
- Nerve kinking due to not mobilizing the nerve far enough proximally or distally during transposition

- Flexion contracture following submuscular transposition
- Elbow instability secondary to excessive resection of medial epicondyle
- Flexor pronator origin avulsion
- Flexor pronator weakness
- Tenderness at the osteotomy site of medial epicondyle
- Nerve adherence to surrounding tissues/scarring (minimized with early mobilization)

REFERENCES

1. Rayan GM, Jensen C, Duke J. Elbow flexion test in the normal population. *J Hand Surg Am.* 1992;17(1):86-89.
2. Siemionow M, Agaoglu G, Hoffmann R. Anatomic characteristics of a fascia and its bands overlying the ulnar nerve in the proximal forearm: a cadaver study. *J Hand Surg Eur.* 2007;32(3):302-307.
3. Goldfarb CA, Sutter MM, Martens EJ, Manske PR. Incidence of re-operation and subjective outcome following in situ decompression of the ulnar nerve at the cubital tunnel. *J Hand Surg Eur.* 2009;34(3):379-383.
4. Dellon AL. Review of treatment results for ulnar nerve entrapment at the elbow. *J Hand Surg Am.* 1989;14: 688-700.
5. Zlowodzki M, Chan S, Bhandari M, Kalliainen L, Schubert W. Anterior transposition compared with simple decompression for treatment of cubital tunnel syndrome. A meta-analysis of randomized, controlled trials. *J Bone Joint Surg Am.* 2007;89:2591-2598.
6. McAdam SA, Gandhi R, Bezuhly M, Lefaivre KA. Simple decompression versus anterior subcutaneous and submuscular transposition of the ulnar nerve for cubital tunnel syndrome: a meta-analysis. *J Hand Surg Am.* 2008;33(8):1314.e1-12.

Relevant Review Articles

Elhassan B, Stteinmann SP. Entrapment neuropathy of the
    ulnar nerve. *J Am Acad Orthop Surg.* 2007;15(11):
    672-681.
Gellman H. Compression of the ulnar nerve at the elbow.
    Instr Course Lect. 2008;57:187-197.

CHAPTER 8

DISTAL BICEPS TENDON RUPTURE

Ryan G. Miyamoto, MD and
Peter J. Millett, MD, MSc

MECHANISM OF INJURY/ PATHOPHYSIOLOGY

Distal biceps ruptures compose approximately 3% of all ruptures of the biceps tendon, and they most commonly occur just proximal to the tendinous insertion onto the bicipital tuberosity. The pathogenesis of distal biceps ruptures is not well understood. Current theories involve both **vascular** and **mechanical** mechanisms as the reason for rupture at the musculotendinous junction.

Seiler and colleagues performed both an anatomic and a radiographic study to help elucidate these mechanisms.[1] The anatomic portion of the study demonstrated a consistent hypovascular zone measuring 2.14 cm proximal to the tendon insertion. The radiographic portion of the study demonstrated that in the pronated position, the space available for the tendon was 48% less than in supination. Additionally, with the forearm in pronation, the biceps tendon occupied 85% of the radioulnar space at the level of the tuberosity, implying a mechanical cause for rupture.

KEY HISTORY POINTS

- Patients with distal biceps tendon ruptures frequently note an unexpected extension force

Rohde RS, Millett PJ, eds.
*Evaluation and Management
of Common Upper Extremity Disorders:
A Practical Handbook* (pp 123-138).
© 2011 Taylor & Francis Group.

applied to a flexed arm followed by an eccentric contraction.

- The resulting acute pain may be sudden, sharp, and described as a "tearing" sensation in the antecubital fossa and posterolateral aspect of the elbow.
- As acute pain subsides, a chronic pain may linger, particularly with activity.
- The patient may report mild weakness with elbow flexion and marked weakness with forearm supination.
- A loss of biceps contour or a "Popeye" deformity may be described by the patient.

KEY EXAMINATION POINTS

Examination findings commonly involved in distal biceps tendon ruptures can include:

- Tenderness to palpation in the antecubital fossa
- Swelling and ecchymosis in the antecubital fossa and along the medial side of the arm, elbow, or forearm
- A loss of biceps contour or a "Popeye" deformity
- A palpable defect in the antecubital fossa
- Significant weakness in forearm supination and elbow flexion compared to the contralateral arm
- Ruland and colleagues developed the biceps squeeze test to help elucidate the integrity of the biceps tendon.[2] Similar to the Thompson test used to aid the diagnosis of an Achilles tendon rupture, the biceps brachii is squeezed to elicit forearm supination if the tendon is intact.
- O'Driscoll and colleagues described the hook test for diagnosis of complete biceps tendon avulsions (Figure 8-1).[3] This test is performed by inserting the finger under the lateral edge of the biceps tendon between the brachialis and biceps tendon and hooking the finger under the cord-like structure spanning the

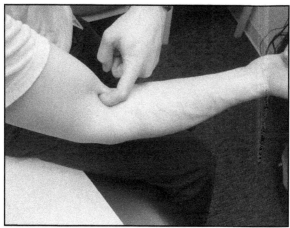

Figure 8-1. Demonstration of the hook test.

antecubital fossa with the patient's elbow flexed at 90 degrees. In a patient with a distal biceps tendon rupture, no structure will be palpated or "hooked." A crucial portion of the test is to hook the lateral edge of the biceps tendon, not the medial side, to prevent mistaking the lacertus fibrosus for an intact biceps tendon.

ADDITIONAL TESTING OR IMAGING

- **Radiographs** of the elbow, including anteroposterior and lateral views, may show some enlargement and irregular changes about the tuberosity or an avulsion of the tuberosity itself.
- **Ultrasound** has been used with varying degrees of success for identifying these injuries but is not routinely obtained.

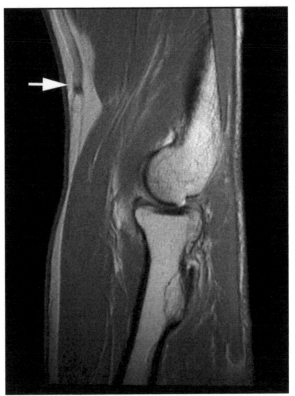

Figure 8-2. MRI of a patient with a distal biceps tendon rupture showing retraction of the torn tendon (white arrow).

- **Magnetic resonance imaging** (MRI) remains the gold standard for identifying these injuries. It can assist in delineating the integrity and any intrasubstance degeneration of the tendon, as well as to determine if a tear is partial-thickness versus full-thickness (Figure 8-2).

- Giuffrè and Moss described the flexed abducted supinated (FABS) position for MRI of the distal biceps.[4] The elbow is flexed to 90 degrees, the shoulder abducted to 180 degrees, and the forearm supinated; this can help one to visualize the full length of the biceps from the musculotendinous junction to the tuberosity insertion.

TREATMENT OPTIONS: NONOPERATIVE

Nonoperative treatment generally is reserved for sedentary patients who do not require elbow flexion and supination strength and endurance or patients not medically fit for surgery.[5]

- Treatment consists of temporary immobilization in a splint and pain control, including the use of nonsteroidal anti-inflammatory drugs.
- Physiotherapy commences once pain is reasonably controlled.
- There is a possibility that some chronic-activity–related arm pain and mild weakness in supination and elbow flexion may result with nonoperative measures.[6]

TREATMENT OPTIONS: OPERATIVE

Surgical treatment for distal biceps tendon ruptures involves anatomic repair of the distal end of the tendon to its insertion on the radial tuberosity. The creation of newer fixation methods and biomechanically stronger implants has caused intense debate about the optimal surgical technique for these injuries. Surgical complications include nerve injuries from paresthesias to palsies, complex regional pain syndrome, heterotopic ossification, radioulnar synostosis, loss of forearm rotation, and wound infection.

Two-Incision Versus One-Incision Repair

Two-Incision

- Boyd and Anderson described their 2-incision technique in 1961, noting a lower rate of nerve injuries as well as a more anatomic reattachment of the tendon through bone tunnels compared to previous 1-incision techniques.[7] Failla and colleagues described a modification of the classic Boyd and Anderson approach involving a limited muscle-splitting approach through the extensor muscle mass in the second incision without exposure of the proximal ulna.[8] Chavan and colleagues performed a systematic review of the literature on 2-incision distal biceps tendon repairs and noted an overall complication rate of 16% (23 of 142 elbows); the majority of these demonstrated a loss of forearm rotation or rotational strength.[9]

One-Incision

- Improvement of alternative fixation methods including suture anchors, interference screws, and EndoButtons (Smith & Nephew, Andover, MA) have made the 1-incision technique a popular option with less incidence of heterotopic ossification than following the 2-incision approach. The meta-analysis performed by Chavan and colleagues analyzing 1-incision distal biceps tendon repairs reported an overall complication rate of 18% (29 of 165 elbows); the most common complication—nerve injury—was reported in 13% of patients.[9]

SURGICAL ANATOMY

- The biceps tendon is composed of 2 heads. It is innervated by a single branch of the musculo-cutaneous nerve 62% of the time at a point 130 mm below the acromion.

- A second branch of the musculocutaneous nerve may be present and innervates the bicep approximately 24 mm distal to this point.

- Distally, the tendon unit inserts onto the bicipital tuberosity on the proximal portion of the radius (Figure 8-3).

- An associated structure, the lacertus fibrosus (bicipital aponeurosis), originates from the distal tendon as it passes anterior to the elbow joint and expands ulnarly, blending with the fascia of the forearm.

- The distal tendon fibers themselves rotate in a predictable pattern as they reach their insertion, clockwise in the left elbow and counterclockwise in the right elbow.

- The anteromedial fibers follow a linear path to their attachment, while the posterolateral fibers coil beneath the medial fibers to their attachment on the tuberosity.

- The distal portion of the short-head contribution of the tendon inserts more distally on the tuberosity where biomechanically it acts as a powerful flexor of the elbow.

- The distal portion of the long-head contribution inserts further from the central axis of the forearm, thereby providing a powerful lever arm for supination.

- The lacertus fibrosus originates at the level of the musculotendinous junction and consists of 3 distinct layers, enveloping the forearm flexor muscles and serving as a stabilizer to the distal tendon.

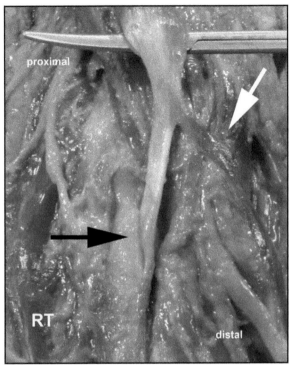

Figure 8-3. Anatomy of the distal biceps tendon insertion (black arrow) to the radial tuberosity; white arrow shows bicipital aponeurosis (lacertus fibrosus).

- The **lateral antebrachial cutaneous nerve** (LACN) has the following characteristics:
    - Is the terminal branch of the musculocutaneous nerve and supplies sensation to the volar lateral aspect of the forearm
    - Pierces the fascia of the arm near the musculotendinous junction of the distal biceps tendon

- □ Must be avoided in the superficial dissection during tendon repairs
- The **posterior interosseous nerve** (PIN) has the following characteristics:
  - □ Is a branch of the radial nerve that divides from the superficial branch anterior to the humeral epicondyle
  - □ Courses on the lateral side of the proximal radius and enters the supinator muscle between its humeral and radial heads
  - □ Is the motor nerve most at risk during 1-incision repairs
  - □ One study evaluating EndoButton-repaired distal tendon ruptures also included cadaveric dissections, which showed an average distance of 9.3 mm from the EndoButton to the PIN and a consistent layer of supinator muscle that interposed between the 2 in all cadavers.[8]

PROCEDURES

Single-incision anatomic reattachment with EndoButton fixation is described because it is currently the senior author's preferred method of fixation.

- Our preferred anesthetic technique is general endotracheal anesthesia or laryngeal mask airway. We do not place a preoperative regional block so that an accurate postoperative neurovascular examination can be performed. A postoperative block may be placed for pain control following documentation of the neurovascular examination prior to discharge home.
- Intravenous antibiotics are administered and the patient is positioned supine with the arm placed on an arm board. A sterile tourniquet is available but is not placed routinely on the arm prior to sterile preparation.

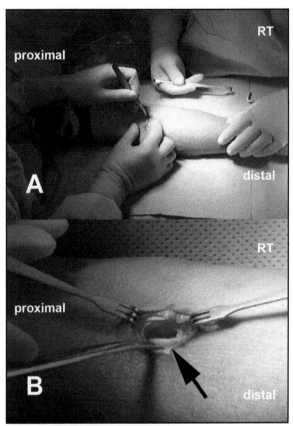

Figure 8-4. Example of a single-incision technique used for distal biceps repair. (A) Incision. (B) Approach with ruptured biceps tendon (black arrow).

- A 4-cm transverse incision is made approximately 2 to 3 cm distal to the elbow crease. A fluoroscopy machine may be used prior to skin incision to help center the incision over the radial tuberosity (Figure 8-4).

- Skin and subcutaneous dissection is performed; care is taken not to injure the LACN.
- The interval between the pronator teres and the brachioradialis is developed to the level of the lacertus fibrosus. A plexus of veins may be present in the interval; this should be identified and hemostasis maintained.
- In acute cases, a hematoma is often present and can be used to help identify the tendon stump in the proximal aspect of the wound.
- Following tendon identification, the frayed end is débrided of any necrotic or degenerative tissue and a running locking stitch with nonabsorbable, heavy, braided suture (No. 2 FiberWire, Arthrex Inc, Naples, FL) is placed starting distally, advancing 2 cm proximally, and then returning distally.
- The EndoButton is secured to the tendon within 2 to 3 mm of the tendon edge so that it may be flipped.
- The radial tuberosity is identified and gentle retraction, particularly on the lateral side of the radius, should be used to avoid injury to the radial nerve or PIN.
- Placement of the Beath pin and subsequent reaming is performed with the forearm in maximal supination to avoid injury to the PIN.
- Care is taken to avoid aiming laterally while drilling because this also could endanger the PIN.
- The wound is irrigated after reaming to remove all bone fragments and to help to prevent heterotopic ossificiation.
- The tendon and EndoButton are passed through the tunnel, the EndoButton is flipped, and fluoroscopy can be used to confirm deployment of the EndoButton (Figure 8-5).
- The skin is closed subcutaneously with 2-0 absorbable suture and a 3-0 running subcuticular stitch. Steri-Strips (3M, St. Paul, MN) are applied and a posterior splint with the elbow in 90 degrees of flexion and neutral rotation is placed.

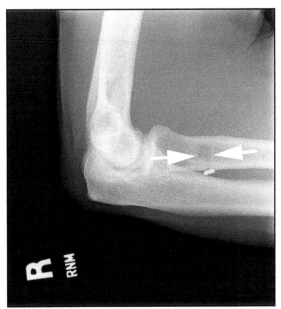

Figure 8-5. Distal biceps tendon repair utilizing a cortical fixation button; white arrows pointing at the socket for the tendon.

REHABILITATION

- There is wide variation in postoperative protocols; improved fixation methods allow earlier range of motion and increasingly aggressive rehabilitation.
- Classically, the arm has been immobilized in flexion with the forearm in a neutral position for a period ranging from 1 to 6 weeks.
- Passive and active assisted range of motion is initiated and gradually progresses with the goal of achieving full extension by week 6.
- Motion and strengthening are increased in intensity after 6 weeks.

OUTCOMES

Surgical Versus Nonsurgical Treatment

- Recently, studies by Chillemi and colleagues and Hetsroni and colleagues showed superior results for subjective functional outcomes and objective outcomes in patients treated operatively for distal biceps tendon ruptures versus their nonoperative counterparts.[10,11] The retrospective review by Freeman and colleagues evaluated 18 patients with unrepaired distal biceps tendon ruptures and compared them to historical controls that had been treated operatively.[6] The mean supination and flexion strengths in the nonoperative cohort were 74% and 88%, respectively, compared to the contralateral arm. Compared to the operatively treated historical cohort, there was a significant difference in supination strength (74% compared to 101%) but not flexion strength (88% compared to 97%).

Two-Incision Versus One-Incision Repair

- El-Hawary and colleagues conducted a prospective study of 9 patients undergoing single-incision suture anchor fixation versus 10 patients undergoing a modified Boyd and Anderson 2-incision technique.[12] At the 1-year mark, the 1-incision group had regained 11.7 more degrees of elbow flexion than the 2-incision group (142.8 degrees versus 131.1 degrees, respectively). However, although at 1-year there were no differences in flexion or supination strength or supination motion, flexion strength returned more rapidly in the 2-incision group. The complication rate in the 1-incision group was 44% (4 of 9 elbows), including 3 LACN paresthesias and 1 case of flexion contracture from heterotopic ossification. In the 2-incision group, the complication rate was 10% (1 of 10); a transient superficial radial nerve paresthesia occurred. Chavan and colleagues conducted a meta-analysis of clinical outcomes with 2-incision versus the 1-incision technique using criteria that included objective strength and motion testing.[9] The authors reported a 69% satisfactory outcome rate (60 of 87 elbows) with the 2-incision group versus a 94% satisfaction rate (135 of 143 elbows) in the 1-incision group; this corresponded to an odds ratio of an unsatisfactory outcome after a 2-incision approach of 7:6. The majority of unsatisfactory outcomes were due to loss of forearm rotation or strength.

Surgical Fixation Methods

- Greenberg and colleagues evaluated the pullout strengths of the Mitek G4 Superanchor (Mitek, Westwood, MA), transosseous tunnels, and the EndoButton.[13] The pullout strength of the EndoButton was 3 times stronger than the bone tunnels and 2 times stronger than the Mitek anchor, thus providing compelling evidence for its use. The superior failure to load of the EndoButton construct also was confirmed in studies by Kettler and colleagues and Mazzocca and colleagues when compared to suture anchors, bone tunnels, and interference screws.[14,15]

POTENTIAL COMPLICATIONS

- Heterotopic ossification with restricted forearm rotation (more common with 2-incision technique)
- Radioulnar synostosis
- PIN palsy (more common with 1-incision technique)
- Sensory nerve paresthesias (LACN, PIN)
- Persistent anterior elbow pain
- Superficial wound infection
- Re-rupture of the tendon
- Complex regional pain syndrome

REFERENCES

1. Seiler JG 3rd, Parker LM, Chamberland PD, Sherbourne GM, Carpenter WA. The distal biceps tendon. Two potential mechanisms involved in its rupture: arterial supply and mechanical impingement. *J Shoulder Elbow Surg*. 1995;4(3):149-156.
2. Ruland RT, Dunbar RP, Bowen JD. The biceps squeeze test for diagnosis of distal biceps tendon ruptures. *Clin Orthop Relat Res*. 2005;437:128-131.
3. O'Driscoll SW, Goncalves LB, Dietz P. The hook test for distal biceps tendon avulsion. *Am J Sports Med*. 2007;35(11):1865-1869.
4. Giuffrè BM, Moss MJ. Optimal positioning for MRI of the distal biceps brachii tendon: flexed abducted supinated view. *AJR Am J Roentgenol*. 2004;182(4):944-946.
5. Ramsey ML. Distal biceps tendon injuries: diagnosis and management. *J Am Acad Orthop Surg*. 1999;7: 199-207.
6. Freeman CR, McCormick KR, Mahoney D, Baratz M, Lubahn JD. Nonoperative treatment of distal biceps tendon ruptures compared with a historical control group. *J Bone Joint Surg Am*. 2009;91:2329-2334.
7. Boyd HB, Anderson LD. A method for reinsertion of the distal biceps brachii tendon. *J Bone Joint Surg Am*. 1961;43:1041-1043.

8. Failla JM, Amadio PC, Morrey BF, Beckenbaugh RD. Proximal radioulnar synostosis after repair of distal biceps brachii rupture by the two-incision technique. Report of four cases. *Clin Orthop Relat Res.* 1990;253:133-136.

9. Chavan PR, Duquin TR, Bisson LJ. Repair of the ruptured distal biceps tendon: a systematic review. *Am J Sports Med.* 2008;36(8):1618-1624.

10. Chillemi C, Marinelli M, De Cupis V. Rupture of the distal biceps brachii tendon: conservative treatment versus anatomic reinsertion—clinical and radiological evaluation after 2 years. *Arch Orthop Trauma Surg.* 2007;127(8): 705-708.

11. Hetsroni I, Pilz-Burstein R, Nyska M, Back Z, Barchilon V, Mann G. Avulsion of the distal biceps brachii tendon in middle-aged population: is surgical repair advisable? A comparative study of 22 patients treated with either nonoperative management or early anatomical repair. *Injury.* 2008;39(7):753-760.

12. El-Hawary R, Macdermid JC, Faber KJ, Patterson SD, King GJ. Distal biceps tendon repair: comparison of surgical techniques. *J Hand Surg Am.* 2003;28(3):496-502.

13. Greenberg JA, Fernandez JJ, Wang T, Turner C. EndoButton-assisted repair of distal biceps tendon ruptures. *J Shoulder Elbow Surg.* 2003;12(5):484-490.

14. Kettler M, Lunger J, Kuhn V, Mutschler W, Tingart MJ. Failure strengths in distal biceps tendon repair. *Am J Sports Med.* 2007;35(9):1544-1548.

15. Mazzocca AD, Burton KJ, Romeo AA, Santangelo S, Adams DA, Arciero RA. Biomechanical evaluation of 4 techniques of distal biceps brachii tendon repair. *Am J Sports Med.* 2007;35(2):252-258.

Relevant Review Articles

Chavan PR, Duquin TR, Bisson LJ. Repair of the ruptured distal biceps tendon: a systematic review. *Am J Sports Med.* 2008;36(8):1618-1624.

CHAPTER 9 | PROXIMAL HUMERUS FRACTURES

Charles J. Petit, MD;
Christopher B. Dewing, MD;
and Peter J. Millett, MD, MSc

MECHANISM OF INJURY/ PATHOPHYSIOLOGY

Proximal humerus fractures are the second most common upper extremity fracture and their incidence is increasing as the population ages. Younger patients typically present after a higher energy injury, while older patients typically present with a fall from standing. The mechanisms of injury are primarily traumatic and include the following types:

Indirect Trauma

- More common
- Fall on outstretched hand or on flexed elbow
  □ Force transferred to proximal humerus
  □ Impaction against glenoid and/or acromion results in fracture
- Electrical shock or seizure
  □ Resulting rotator cuff contraction may avulse greater tuberosity

Rohde RS, Millett PJ, eds.
Evaluation and Management
of Common Upper Extremity Disorders:
A Practical Handbook (pp 139-160).
© 2011 Taylor & Francis Group.

Direct Trauma

- Less common
- Direct impact against proximal humerus leads to fracture
- Fracture configuration is determined by the following factors:
    - Position of the proximal humerus at time of fall
    - Bone quality of proximal humerus (often osteopenic or osteoporotic in elderly)
    - Pull of rotator cuff muscles on greater and lesser tuberosities
    - Pull of extrinsic muscles (deltoid, pectoralis major)

KEY HISTORY POINTS

- History of traumatic injury (eg, fall)
- Symptoms including shoulder pain, swelling, and bruising
- Identify additional injuries in affected shoulder, particularly rotator cuff tears
- Determine whether there is a known history of osteoporosis (consider referral for bone mineral density testing if needed)
- In elderly patients, assess for syncope as a cause of falling

KEY EXAMINATION POINTS

- Evaluate head, neck, and chest for injury.
- Inspect skin integrity to rule out open fracture.
- Evaluate sensation in axillary, median, radial, and ulnar nerve distributions.
- Grade motor function of muscles innervated by the axillary, median, radial, and ulnar nerves.

- Evaluate extremity vascular status.
- Assess swelling and echymosis; remove bracelets and rings.

ADDITIONAL TESTING OR IMAGING

Adequate imaging is necessary to classify and treat a proximal humerus fracture properly. Plain radiographs are essential. When questions exist regarding the number of fracture fragments and displacement, further imaging with a computed tomography (CT) scan is warranted. Magnetic resonance imaging (MRI) does not offer the osseous detail of CT scan.

- Radiographs
  - □ True anteroposterior view of glenohumeral joint
  - □ Scapular Y view
  - □ Axillary view (must be obtained to rule out fracture-dislocation)
- CT scan
  - □ Thin slice with coronal and sagittal reformats
  - □ Three-dimensional reconstructions can be helpful if available
- MRI
  - □ May be considered in preoperative planning for the management of proximal humerus fractures in rotator cuff-deficient patients

Fracture Classification

The most widely used classification is the Neer classification. The proximal humerus is divided into 4 parts: the humeral head, humeral shaft, greater tuberosity, and lesser tuberosity. Displacement is defined as angulation greater than 45 degrees or displacement greater than 1 cm. Parts are defined by displacement, not the presence of fracture lines; a 1-part fracture may have multiple fracture lines but no displaced fragments (Figure 9-1).

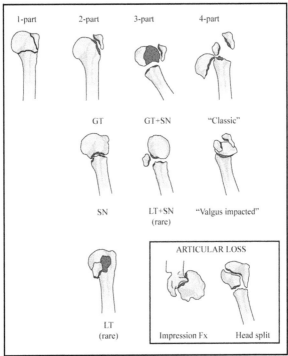

Figure 9-1. Neer classification illustrated. (Adapted from Bucholz RW, Heckman JD, Court-Brown C, Tornetta P, Koval KJ, Wirth MA, eds. *Rockwood and Green's Fractures in Adults*. 6th ed. Philadelphia, PA: Lippincott Williams and Wilkins; 2005.)

TREATMENT OPTIONS: NONOPERATIVE

- Nonoperative treatment is indicated in the case of nondisplaced or minimally displaced fractures (less than 1 cm of displacement and less than 45 degrees of angulation), displaced fractures in patients with low functional demands or with major medical comorbidities, or greater tuberosity fractures with less than 5 cm of displacement.

- The arm is immobilized in a sling for 2 to 3 weeks. Early hand, wrist, and elbow range of motion exercise is encouraged.
- Gentle passive range of motion exercise begins at 2 to 3 weeks. Radiographs are repeated 2 weeks after injury to ensure no further displacement and again following beginning range of motion exercise.
- If displacement or significant pain is noted with range of motion exercise, additional immobilization for 2 to 3 weeks is followed by repeat radiographs.
- Active range of motion begins at 6 weeks or when early callus is noted on radiographs.
- Strengthening begins at 10 to 12 weeks after injury.

TREATMENT OPTIONS: OPERATIVE

As detailed below, there are numerous options for the treatment of proximal humerus fractures.

General Indications

- Fractures with more than 1 cm of displacement or more than 45 degrees of angulation
- Greater tuberosity fractures with more than 5 mm of superior displacement
- Minimally displaced fractures in polytrauma patient to facilitate early mobility

Goals

- Restoration of proximal humerus anatomy
- Minimal disruption of blood supply to proximal humerus

Decision Making

- In general, there is little agreement between surgeons on when to apply specific operative techniques to particular fracture patterns.[1]
- Current decision making is best guided by an assessment of the patient's age, activity level, fracture pattern, humeral head perfusion, and overall bone quality.
- Humeral head ischemia has been shown to be highly associated with articular fractures at the anatomic neck with displacement of the medial hinge greater than 2 mm.[2,3]
- Combined medial and lateral cortical thickness of more than 4 mm should allow for successful open reduction and internal fixation (ORIF), while less than 4 mm might necessitate arthroplasty or suture fixation.[4]

SURGICAL ANATOMY

The deltopectoral approach is the most commonly used approach for open treatment of proximal humerus (Figure 9-2) fractures. Other approaches such as the transdeltoid have been described but are beyond the scope of this book.

- The incision extends from the coracoid process proximally to the deltoid tuberosity of the humerus distally.
- The cephalic vein marks the internervous plane between the deltoid and the pectoralis major.
- Due to the need for lateral exposure, the cephalic vein is most easily retracted medially with the pectoralis.
- The deltoid is retracted laterally and the pectoralis medially by a self-retaining retractor or an assistant.

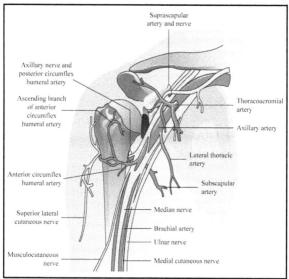

Figure 9-2. Neurovascular anatomy surrounding the proximal humerus. (Adapted from Bucholz RW, Heckman JD, Court-Brown C, Tornetta P, Koval KJ, Wirth MA, eds. *Rockwood and Green's Fractures in Adults*. 6th ed. Philadelphia, PA: Lippincott Williams and Wilkins; 2005.)

- The biceps groove is identified and dissection around it is minimized to prevent damage to the ascending branch of the anterior humeral circumflex artery.
- If the bicipital groove is significantly damaged and cannot be anatomically reconstructed, biceps tenodesis should be performed.
- Exposure can be enhanced with release of the superior portion of the pectoralis tendon and with partial release of the deltoid from the humerus.
- The superior portion of the pectoralis insertion should be marked prior to any release because it

can serve as a landmark for humeral head height. The average distance from the superior-most aspect of the humeral head to the proximal pectoralis insertion is 5.6 cm.[5]

PROCEDURES

Closed Reduction Percutaneous Pinning

- Operative indications: Greater than 1 cm of displacement between head and shaft or 5 mm of displacement of greater tuberosity
- Contraindications include severely osteopenic or osteoporotic bone and noncompliant patients. Medial calcar comminution is a relative contraindication.[6,7]
- May be utilized for isolated greater tuberosity fractures or 2-, 3-, or 4-part fractures.[7-9]
- The patient is positioned in a beach chair at 45 degrees.
- The surgeon confirms that the C-arm can be maneuvered easily with the arc over the operative shoulder and that appropriate anteroposterior and axillary lateral views are obtainable (Figure 9-3).
- Reduction is achieved by initial axial traction and completed with abduction, translation, and rotation as needed.
- In 3- or 4-part fractures, reduction is aided by percutaneously placing an instrument in the subacromial space to manipulate fracture fragments.
- Pin placement requires attention to correct starting position and neurovascular anatomy.
  - Typically, three or four 2.8-mm Kirschner wires are placed from distal to proximal through small skin incisions, allowing the surgeon to

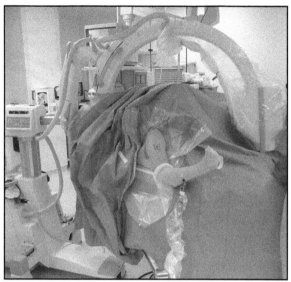

Figure 9-3. Operative setup for fixation of proximal humerus fractures.

protect the axillary nerve by spreading with a hemostat to the starting position on the cortex of the humerus. Additional pins or percutaneous screws may be placed from proximal to distal across the greater tuberosity and into the medial cortex distal to the neck fracture.

□ For 3- and 4-part fractures, additional pins or screws might be necessary to stabilize the lesser tuberosity fragment.

□ Care must be taken to avoid articular penetration and to avoid all pins crossing the fracture at the same level, compromising rotational stability of the construct.

□ Studies have shown that the biceps tendon and axillary nerve are at risk.[10,11]

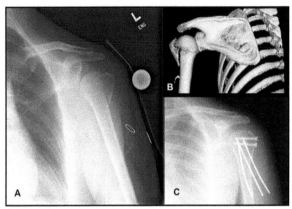

Figure 9-4. (A) and (B) Preoperative radiographs and 3-D CT scan of a valgus-impacted 3-part fracture with displaced humeral head and greater tuberosity fragments. (C) Postoperative radiograph showing reduced fracture and placement of 2 percutaneous screws and 3 percutaneous pins.

- Percutaneous screw fixation can be achieved over the provisional Kirschner wires if desired; specific systems are commercially available.
- Pins should be cut at a length sufficient to allow skin closure but enable easy retrieval, typically 3 to 4 weeks postoperatively (Figure 9-4).

Open Reduction and Internal Fixation With Locking Plate

- A standard deltopectoral approach is required.
- Careful palpation and elevation of the axillary nerve is critical when placing the plate against the proximal humeral shaft.
- C-arm positioning is as described previously for percutaneous fixation (see Figure 9-3).

- Meticulous exposure of the principal fracture lines will facilitate fracture reduction.
- Sutures through the rotator cuff tendons may assist in obtaining reduction and ultimately can be tied to the plate through available suture holes.
- Provisional Kirschner wire fixation may be used to maintain reduction of the major fracture fragments while plate position is optimized.
- Plate position is critical. The implant should abut directly the lateral cortex of the humerus and be distal enough to avoid impingement when the shoulder is abducted; the proximal aspect usually is 8 mm distal to the tip of the greater tuberosity.
- Locking plates have demonstrated biomechanical properties superior to standard plates or blade plate constructs, particularly in the setting of medial comminution and/or osteoporotic bone.[12,13]
- If significant medial comminution is present, calcar-specific screws are necessary.[14]
- Beware of articular screw penetration. Obtain final live fluoroscopic views with the shoulder in internal and external rotation to confirm screw placement (Figure 9-5).

Hemiarthroplasty

- Indications include 3- and 4-part fractures, fracture-dislocations in osteoporotic bone, or head-splitting fractures with more than 40% involvement of the articular surface.
- Contraindications include active infection and severe rotator cuff deficiency.
- A standard deltopectoral approach, as described previously, is used.
- Sutures should be placed at the bone-tendon interface at both lesser and greater tuberosities to enhance control of the tuberosities.

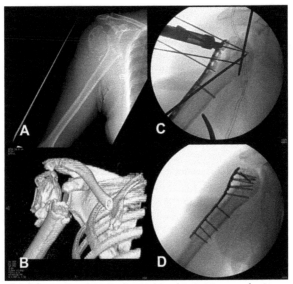

Figure 9-5. (A) and (B) Radiograph and 3-D CT scan of a 3-part fracture-dislocation of the proximal humerus. (C) Intraoperative fluoroscopy showing placement of plate and maintenance of reduction with Kirschner wires. (D) Final intraoperative fluoroscopy view.

- The head fragments should be removed and the glenoid inspected to ensure no glenoid fixation or component is needed.
- The shaft must be prepared carefully and specific attention to height and retroversion is required. The bicipital groove is a helpful landmark for version and typically the head to tuberosity distance should be 8 mm.[15,16]
- Use of cement is based on surgeon preference and bone quality. Tuberosity repair may be augmented by bone graft.

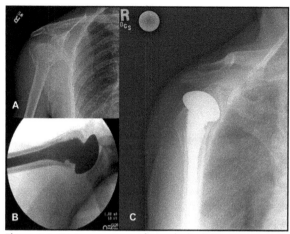

Figure 9-6. (A) Preoperative radiograph displaying 4-part proximal humerus fracture. (B) Intraoperative fluoroscopy after placement of hemiarthroplasty. (C) Postoperative radiograph.

- Anatomic repair of the tuberosities should be achieved to maximize functional outcome.[17]
- Augmenting the tuberosity repair with cerclage sutures passed about the stem prior to insertion will increase the strength of the repair (Figure 9-6).

Intramedullary Fixation

Intramedullary fixation is beyond the scope of this book. It is indicated primarily for unstable 2-part fractures and favored for minimally invasive technique when compared to open plate fixation. Familiarity with specific implant systems is essential. Intramedullary fixation has been shown to be biomechanically less stable than locked plating.[18] It is technically challenging to maintain reduction during nail insertion, and additional pins may be necessary to prevent varus alignment of the proximal fragment.[19]

Open Reduction and Internal Fixation With Alternative Fixation (Suture Fixation)

This technique relies on viable rotator cuff tendons to achieve fracture reduction and stabilization. It is contra-indicated for treatment of fractures older than 6 weeks.[6] Drill holes are placed at greater tuberosity, lesser tuber-osity, and on the neck distal to the fracture, facilitating suture passage and fixation. The biceps tendon must be tenodesed or carefully avoided during suture passage.

Reverse Total Shoulder Arthroplasty

The technical aspects of reverse total shoulder arthroplasty are beyond the scope of this chapter. Reverse total shoulder arthroplasty should be considered in cases of failed hemiarthroplasty or in the delayed treatment of high-grade proximal humerus fractures in the setting of osteoporotic bone and rotator cuff deficiency. No inter-mediate or long-term results have been published at the time of this printing.

REHABILITATION

- Rehabilitation protocols must be tailored to the patient, the fracture pattern, and the quality of the reduction and fixation or arthroplasty.
- In general, percutaneous fixation with Kirschner wires left buried beneath the skin should be treated with complete sling immobilization and gentle pen-dulum exercises only until Kirschner wire removal

at 4 to 6 weeks. Passive and active range of motion may be started thereafter, provided the fracture was stable at the time of Kirschner wire removal.

- Patients treated by ORIF or hemiarthroplasty should undergo initial sling immobilization for 10 to 14 days. Supervised passive range of motion may begin immediately if stable fixation was achieved, active motion may begin 4 weeks postoperatively, and strengthening may start at 6 weeks.
- Follow-up radiographs should be taken at weeks 2 and 6, then at 3-month intervals. Osteonecrosis has been documented as late as 6 to 12 months postoperatively.

OUTCOMES

Nonoperative Treatment

- Minimally displaced fractures have been shown to have 80% good to excellent results.[20]
- Eighty percent good to excellent results have been reported for valgus-impacted fractures.[21]
- In a comparison between operative and nonoperative treatment of translated 2-part proximal humerus fractures, Court-Brown et al found no difference in outcome between operative and nonoperative treatment modalities in elderly patients.[22]

Operative Treatment

Closed Reduction Percutaneous Pinning

- Outcomes have been favorable in most series, with revision rates of 7% to 14%.[6]
- Resch et al reported on the treatment of 27 patients with 3- and 4-part fractures treated with CRPP and found good results for valgus-impacted fracture;

significantly translated 4-part fractures had a 40% (2 of 5) rate of revision to hemiarthroplasty.[9]

■ Fenichel and colleagues found good to excellent results in 70% of 2- and 3-part fractures treated with CRPP. Tuberosity fractures fared worse than neck fractures, and 6% of patients required revision surgery.[23]

Open Reduction and Internal Fixation With Suture Fixation

■ Outcomes have been excellent for isolated greater tuberosity fractures[24] and have been good to excellent in greater than 75% of patients with 2- or 3-part fractures in the largest of series.[25]

Open Reduction and Internal Fixation With Locking Plate

■ Kettler and colleagues reported significantly better results when anatomic reduction of the greater tuberosity is performed and maintained.[26]

■ Gardner and colleagues demonstrated that anatomic reduction of the medial cortex significantly affects the magnitude of subsequent reduction loss.[16]

■ Results of locking-plate fixation are much better for 2- and 3-part fractures than for 4-part fractures.[27]

■ ORIF of head-splitting fractures is not successful.[26]

Hemiarthroplasty

■ Most patients experience significant pain relief.[19,28,29]

■ Two separate studies have shown that tuberosity malposition negatively affects functional results.[19,30]

■ Outcomes frequently are compromised by continued pain and overall poor range of motion.[31]

POTENTIAL COMPLICATIONS

Nonoperative Treatment

- Nonunion
- Malunion

Operative Treatment

- Infection (inherent risk of all operative techniques)
- Nonunion (inherent risk of all fracture fixation techniques)
- Loss of reduction (inherent risk of all fracture fixation techniques)
- Hardware failure (inherent risk of all fracture fixation techniques)
- Pin migration (closed reduction percutaneous pinning)
- Chronic shoulder pain due to violation of rotator cuff upon entry (intramedullary nail fixation)
- Screw perforation of humeral head (noted in 14% in a large series[14]) (ORIF with plate)
- Plate impingement (ORIF with plate)
- Avascular necrosis of humeral head (ORIF with plate)
- Stiffness (ORIF with plate)
- Additional risks of hemiarthroplasty:
    - Tuberosity nonunion or malunion (hemi-arthroplasty)
    - Malpositioning of humeral component (height and version)
    - Implant loosening
    - Intraoperative fracture
    - Instability
    - Glenoid erosion
    - Stiffness

REFERENCES

1. Petit CJ, Millett PJ, Endres NK, Diller D, Harris MB, Warner JJ. Management of proximal humeral fractures: surgeons don't agree. *J Shoulder Elbow Surg.* 2009;19(3): 446-451.
2. Hertel R, Hempfing A, Stiehler M, Leunig M. Predictors of humeral head ischemia after intracapsular fracture of the proximal humerus. *J Shoulder Elbow Surg.* 2004;13(4): 427-433.
3. Nho SJ, Brophy RH, Barker JU, Cornell CN, MacGillivray JD. Innovations in the management of displaced proximal humerus fractures. *J Am Acad Orthop Surg.* 2007;15(1): 12-26.
4. Tingart MJ, Apreleva M, von Stechow D, Zurakowski D, Warner JJ. The cortical thickness of the proximal humeral diaphysis predicts bone mineral density of the proximal humerus. *J Bone Joint Surg Br.* 2003;85(4): 611-617.
5. Murachovsky J, Ikemoto RY, Nascimento LG, Fujiki EN, Milani C, Warner JJ. Pectoralis major tendon reference (PMT): a new method for accurate restoration of humeral length with hemiarthroplasty for fracture. *J Shoulder Elbow Surg.* 2006;15(6):675-678.
6. Nho SJ, Brophy RH, Barker JU, Cornell CN, MacGillivray JD. Management of proximal humeral fractures based on current literature. *J Bone Joint Surg Am.* 2007;89(Suppl 3):44-58.
7. Millett PJ, Warner JJP. Percutaneous treatment of proximal humerus fractures. In: Wirth MA, ed. *Monograph Series 30: Proximal Humerus Fractures.* Rosemont, IL: American Academy of Orthopaedic Surgeons; 2005:15-26.
8. Jaberg H, Warner JJ, Jakob RP. Percutaneous stabilization of unstable fractures of the humerus. *J Bone Joint Surg Am.* 1992;74(4):508-515.
9. Resch H, Povacz P, Frohlich R, Wambacher M. Percutaneous fixation of three- and four-part fractures of the proximal humerus. *J Bone Joint Surg Br.* 1997;79(2):295-300.
10. Rowles DJ, McGrory JE. Percutaneous pinning of the proximal part of the humerus: an anatomic study. *J Bone Joint Surg Am.* 2001;83-A(11):1695-1699.

11. Kamineni S, Ankem H, Sanghavi S. Anatomical considerations for percutaneous proximal humeral fracture fixation. *Injury*. 2004;35(11):1133-1136.

12. Sudkamp N, Bayer J, Hepp P, et al. Open reduction and internal fixation of proximal humeral fractures with use of the locking proximal humerus plate: results of a prospective, multicenter, observational study. *J Bone Joint Surg Am*. 2009;91(6):1320-1328.

13. Siffri PC, Peindl RD, Coley ER, Norton J, Connor PM, Kellam JF. Biomechanical analysis of blade plate versus locking plate fixation for a proximal humerus fracture: comparison using cadaveric and synthetic humeri. *J Orthop Trauma*. 2006;20(8):547-554.

14. Gardner MJ, Weil Y, Barker JU, Kelly BT, Helfet DL, Lorich DG. The importance of medial support in locked plating of proximal humerus fractures. *J Orthop Trauma*. 2007;21(3):185-191.

15. Frankle MA, Ondrovic LE, Markee BA, Harris ML, Lee WE 3rd. Stability of tuberosity reattachment in proximal humeral hemiarthroplasty. *J Shoulder Elbow Surg*. 2002;11(5):413-420.

16. Balg F, Boulianne M, Boileau P. Bicipital groove orientation: considerations for the retroversion of a prosthesis in fractures of the proximal humerus. *J Shoulder Elbow Surg*. 2006;15(2):195-198.

17. Kralinger F, Schwaiger R, Wambacher M, et al. Outcome after primary hemiarthroplasty for fracture of the head of the humerus. A retrospective multicentre study of 167 patients. *J Bone Joint Surg Br*. 2004;86(2):217-219.

18. Edwards SL, Wilson NA, Zhang LQ, Flores S, Merk BR. Two-part surgical neck fractures of the proximal part of the humerus. A biomechanical evaluation of two fixation techniques. *J Bone Joint Surg Am*. 2006;88(10):2258-2264.

19. Agel J, Jones CB, Sanzone AG, Camuso M, Henley MB. Treatment of proximal humeral fractures with polarus nail fixation. *J Shoulder Elbow Surg*. 2004;13(2):191-195.

20. Koval KJ, Gallagher MA, Marsicano JG, Cuomo F, McShinawy A, Zuckerman JD. Functional outcome after minimally displaced fractures of the proximal part of the humerus. *J Bone Joint Surg Am*. 1997;79(2):203-207.

21. Court-Brown CM, Cattermole H, McQueen MM. Impacted valgus fractures (B1.1) of the proximal humerus the results of nonoperative treatment. *J Bone Joint Surg Br.* 2002;84(4):504-508.

22. Court-Brown CM, Garg A, McQueen MM. The translated two-part fracture of the proximal humerus: epidemiology and outcome in the older patient. *J Bone Joint Surg Br.* 2001;83(6):799-804.

23. Fenichel I, Oran A, Burstein G, Perry Pritsch M. Percutaneous pinning using threaded pins as a treatment option for unstable two- and three-part fractures of the proximal humerus: a retrospective study. *Int Orthop.* 2006;30(3):153-157.

24. Flatow EL, Cuomo F, Maday MG, Miller SR, McIlveen SJ, Bigliani LU. Open reduction and internal fixation of two-part displaced fractures of the greater tuberosity of the proximal part of the humerus. *J Bone Joint Surg Am.* 1991;73(8):1213-1218.

25. Park MC, Murthi AM, Roth NS, Blaine TA, Levine WN, Bigliani LU. Two-part and three-part fractures of the proximal humerus treated with suture fixation. *J Orthop Trauma.* 2003;17(5):319-325.

26. Kettler M, Biberthaler P, Braunstein V, Zeiler C, Kroetz M, Mutschler W. Treatment of proximal humeral fractures with the PHILOS angular stable plate. Presentation of 225 cases of dislocated fractures. *Unfallchirurg.* 2006;109(12):1032-1040.

27. Thanasas C, Kontakis G, Angoules A, Limb D, Giannoudis P. Treatment of proximal humerus fractures with locking plates: a systematic review. *J Shoulder Elbow Surg.* 2009;18(6):837-844.

28. Mighell MA, Kolm GP, Collinge CA, Frankle MA. Outcomes of hemiarthroplasty for fractures of the proximal humerus. *J Shoulder Elbow Surg.* 2003;12(6):569-577.

29. Prakash U, McGurty DW, Dent JA. Hemiarthroplasty for severe fractures of the proximal humerus. *J Shoulder Elbow Surg.* 2002;11(5):428-430.

30. Boileau P, Krishnan SG, Tinsi L, Walch G, Coste JS, Mole D. Tuberosity malposition and migration: reasons for poor outcomes after hemiarthroplasty for displaced fractures of the proximal humerus. *J Shoulder Elbow Surg.* 2002;11(5):401-412.

31. Robinson CM, Page RS, Hill RM, Sanders DL, Court-Brown CM, Wakefield AE. Primary hemiarthroplasty for treatment of proximal humeral fractures. *J Bone Joint Surg Am.* 2003;85-A(7):1215-1223.

Relevant Review Articles

Nho SJ, Brophy RH, Barker JU, Cornell CN, MacGillivray JD. Innovations in the management of displaced proximal humerus fractures. *J Am Acad Orthop Surg.* 2007; 15(1):12-26.

Nho SJ, Brophy RH, Barker JU, Cornell CN, MacGillivray JD. Management of proximal humeral fractures based on current literature. *J Bone Joint Surg Am.* 2007;89 (Suppl 3):44-58.

CHAPTER 10 | ACROMIOCLAVICULAR JOINT DISORDERS

Christopher J. Lenarz, MD;
Hinrich J. D. Heuer;
James J. Guerra, MD, FACS; and
Reuben Gobezie, MD

MECHANISM OF INJURY/ PATHOPHYSIOLOGY

Degenerative arthrosis and instability are the most common etiologies of symptoms associated with the acromioclavicular (AC) joint. Degeneration of the fibrocartilaginous disk leads to arthrosis of this joint and is most commonly idiopathic but can be associated with occupational or recreational activities involving repetitive overhead movements. Instability of the AC joint is secondary to a direct or indirect traumatic injury to the articulation, its joint capsule, ligaments, and stabilizing structures (coracoclavicular [CC] ligaments). Instability is graded from I to VI and is based on the distance between the coracoid and the clavicle, the appearance of the AC joint, and the direction of displacement. Chronic instability can lead to arthrosis. Distal clavicle osteolysis also can be seen in weightlifters.

Rohde RS, Millett PJ, eds.
Evaluation and Management
of Common Upper Extremity Disorders:
A Practical Handbook (pp 161-184).
© 2011 Taylor & Francis Group.

KEY HISTORY POINTS

- History of trauma
- Occupational or recreational activities involving repetitive overhead movements
- Pain with overhead activities
- Pain with shoulder adduction

KEY EXAMINATION POINTS

- Tenderness with palpation and manipulation of the AC joint
- Evaluation of stability of the AC joint on direct manipulation
- Reducibility of the AC joint in subluxation or dislocation
- Cross-body adduction test: The arm is flexed forward to the horizontal plane and then passively adducted across the patient's chest; if pain is elicited at the AC joint, the maneuver is positive
- Diagnostic direct injection with local anesthetic of choice

ADDITIONAL TESTING OR IMAGING

- **Radiographs** including anteroposterior (AP) shoulder, Zanca, and axillary views provide useful information. The AP radiograph should be taken at 66% penetration of a standard AP shoulder radiograph to improve visualization of the AC joint and surrounding osseous structures. The Zanca view is taken in the AP plane with a 15-degree cephalic tilt, focusing on the AC joint. Using 50% of the standard voltage of an AP shoulder radiograph improves visualization of the AC joint. The axillary view allows additional evaluation of any anteroposterior translation of the clavicle in relation to the acromion.

Acromioclavicular Joint Injury Grading (Rockwood Classification) (Figure 10-1)

- Grade I—AC ligament sprain without disruption of the CC ligaments or the deltopectoral or trapezial fascia. Radiographic appearance is normal.
- Grade II—AC ligaments are disrupted with a sprain of the CC ligaments. The CC distance is increased less than 25%.
- Grade III—The AC and CC ligaments are disrupted as well as the deltopectoral and trapezial fascia. The CC distance is increased 25% to 100%.
- Grade IV—The AC and CC ligaments and delto-pectoral and trapezial fascia are disrupted. The clavicle is displaced posteriorly, often into the trapezius. This is best visualized on the axillary radiograph. The CC distance is increased.
- Grade V—The AC and CC ligaments are dis-rupted. The deltopectoral and trapezial fascia are more significantly disrupted. The CC distance is increased more than 100%.
- Grade VI—The AC and CC ligaments are dis-rupted as well as the deltopectoral and trapezial fascia. The CC distance is decreased secondary to a caudad displacement of the clavicle to a sub-acromial or subcoracoid position.
- **Magnetic resonance imaging** (MRI) will show edema and inflammation in the AC joint that might be associated with arthrosis. It also can provide information regarding the condition of the soft-tissue structures supporting the joint. Lastly, MRI can be used to identify any concomitant pathology in the rotator cuff, labrum, or other sur-rounding structures.

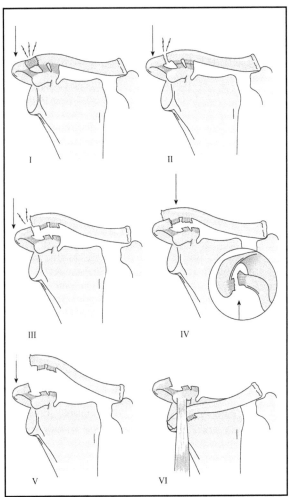

Figure 10-1. Classification of acromioclavicular injuries. (Adapted from Ponce B, Millett PJ, Warner JJP. Acromioclavicular joint instability: reconstruction indications and techniques. *Operative Techniques in Sports Medicine*. 2004;1[12]:35-42.)

TREATMENT OPTIONS: NONOPERATIVE

Degenerative Arthrosis and Distal Clavicle Osteolysis

- Activity modification, including avoidance or modification of activities causing or exacerbating symptoms (eg, weightlifting)
- Oral agents—Nonsteroidal anti-inflammatory drugs (NSAIDs)
- Steroid injections—An intra-articular injection of local anesthetic and corticosteroid[1]

Instability

- Conservative measures including rest and NSAIDs are the standard of care for grades I and II injuries. Currently, the management of grade III injuries is controversial and is the subject of ongoing investigation. Previously, nonoperative care was considered superior; however, with the advent of newer reconstructive and arthroscopic techniques, superior outcomes using operative treatment of these injuries have been suggested.[2]
- Conservative measures for grades IV to VI injuries are indicated only in the patient with significant medical comorbidities in which surgery would pose unnecessary risk.

TREATMENT OPTIONS: OPERATIVE

Degenerative Arthrosis and Distal Clavicle Osteolysis

- Open distal clavicle resection (Mumford procedure)
    - Resection of 0.5 to 1 cm of distal clavicle is performed; resection of the CC ligaments leads to instability and is avoided.
    - Repair of the AC ligaments and deltopectoral fascia helps to prevent horizontal instability.
- Arthroscopic distal clavicle resection
    - This can be performed in conjunction with a subacromial decompression or through a superior approach without a significant violation of the subacromial bursa.
    - Violation of the CC ligaments with excessive clavicle resection introduces the risk of instability.

Instability

- A hook plate with or without CC reconstruction has been used to stabilize AC dislocation.
- Stabilization of the clavicle to the coracoid using screw fixation, suture fixation, or other commercially available fixation techniques has been described. This usually is performed in combination with a soft-tissue reconstructive technique.
- Transfer of the coracoacromial (CA) ligament from the deep portion of the acromion to the distal tip of the clavicle was first described by Weaver and Dunn.[3] The clavicle also is stabilized to the coracoid using one of the aforementioned techniques.
- CC ligament reconstruction using autograft or allograft tendon has been described.[4-7] This can be supplemented by stabilization techniques

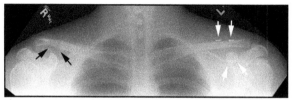

Figure 10-2. X-ray showing 2 cortical fixation button devices on the left (white arrows) and an anatomical coracoclavicular ligament reconstruction using an allograft on the right side (black arrows).

incorporating commercially available suture augmentation devices (Figure 10-2).

SURGICAL ANATOMY

The AC joint is a diarthrodial joint composed of the articulation of the clavicle and scapula with an interposed fibrocartilaginous disk. The joint is encapsulated by stout ligaments that provide primary stability in the anterior and posterior plane. Joint stability is augmented in the cephalad-caudad plane via the trapezoid and conoid ligaments, which attach from the coracoid process to the lateral and medial distal clavicle, respectively. All contribute to the superior shoulder suspensory complex. Dynamic stabilizers of the AC joint include the anterior deltoid muscle and the investing trapezius fascia.

PROCEDURES

Open Distal Clavicle Excision

- The patient is placed in the beach chair or lateral decubitus position and the free upper extremity is prepared and draped. Inclusion of the chest wall in the surgical field is recommended when the clavicle is approached to allow access to major vasculature if necessary.

- An incision is marked centered over the AC joint, extending approximately 2 cm proximal and distal to the joint, along the longitudinal axis of the clavicle.
- Local anesthetic can be administered per surgeon preference.
- An incision is made and the AC joint capsule is exposed using gentle soft-tissue dissection.
- The AC joint capsule is incised in line with the skin incision and the AC joint is exposed in the anterior and posterior directions. Attempts should be made to maintain the capsule integrity to allow for repair prior to closure; this enhances horizontal stability of the remaining distal clavicle.
- The fibrocartilaginous disk is identified and removed using sharp dissection and a rongeur.
- The distal clavicle is marked 0.5 to 1 cm medial to the AC joint, denoting the anticipated location of clavicle excision.
- A sagittal saw is used to remove this segment of bone; care is taken not to remove more than 1 cm of distal clavicle.
- The wound is irrigated and the stability of the clavicle in the cephalad-caudad direction is evaluated.
- The AC capsule and skin are closed.

Arthroscopic Distal Clavicle Resection (With Subacromial Decompression)

- The patient is placed in the beach chair or lateral decubitus position, depending on surgeon preference. The arm and shoulder are prepared and draped sterilely.

- The bony landmarks for determination of portal placement are outlined.
- Arthroscopic examination begins. (Please see Chapters 11 through 14 for descriptions of possible concomitant pathologies.) After the glenohumeral joint is inspected, the arthroscope is placed through the posterolateral portal into the subacromial space.
- Bursal material in the subacromial space is débrided through a midlateral portal, and the rotator cuff is inspected for any pathology that might need to be addressed.
- Following subacromial decompression (see Chapter 11), the AC joint is identified.
- The inferior capsule of the AC joint is resected and an anterior working portal is created in line with the AC joint.
- Depending on the orientation of the AC joint, a portion of the medial acromial facet can be resected to allow greater visualization of the distal clavicle.
- Eight to 10 mm of distal clavicle is resected from posterior to anterior and from inferior to superior. The arthroscope can be placed in either the posterior or lateral portal to improve visualization of the distal clavicle.
- A consistent length of clavicle is resected from the inferior margin to the superior and the integrity of the superior AC joint capsule is maintained.
- Meticulous hemostasis is maintained throughout the procedure and the skin portal is closed with nylon sutures.

Arthroscopic Distal Clavicle Resection (Superior Approach)

- The patient is placed in the beach chair or lateral decubitus position, depending on surgeon preference.

The arm and shoulder are prepared and draped sterilely.

- The bony landmarks for determination of portal placement are outlined.
- The AC joint is localized using small-gauge needles to delineate the location of the fibrocartilaginous disk and the anterior and posterior margins of the AC joint.
- The joint is insufflated with saline solution through the localizing needle.
- Anterior-superior and posterior-superior portals are made in line with the AC joint.
- A small arthroscope is placed into the anterior portal and a small-diameter shaver is introduced into the posterior portal.
- The joint is débrided of the fibrocartilaginous disk material as well as any other intra-articular debris. The AC joint capsule is maintained.
- A small burr is introduced through the working portal, and the distal clavicle resection is completed in a linear fashion beginning on the superior-posterior border of the distal clavicle and progressing anteriorly as far as can be visualized.
- Instruments in the working and visualization portals can be interchanged, allowing visualization of the anterior clavicle; this enables resection of the remaining anterior portion through the anterior portal.
- Resection continues until the AC joint space is approximately 1 cm. Meticulous hemostasis is maintained. The portals are closed using nylon suture.

Modified Weaver-Dunn Procedure (Coracoacromial Ligament Transfer)

- General anesthesia is induced with an interscalene block if that is an option. The patient is placed into the beach chair position. The operative upper extremity is prepared and draped sterilely.

- The borders of the clavicle and acromion are outlined. A longitudinal incision is made along the clavicle; this extends laterally onto the anterior border of the acromion.

- The anterior edge of the deltoid is elevated from the anterior medial acromion and the distal third of the clavicle and retracted anteriorly.

- The clavicle is exposed and a 1-cm segment of the distal clavicle is resected using an oscillating saw. Beveling the distal end of the clavicle from superior-lateral to inferior-medial will increase exposure of cancellous bone to allow attachment of the CA ligament.

- A 0.5-cm wafer of the acromion is resected with an oscillating saw to detach the CA ligament; this cut is beveled in the superior-medial to inferior-lateral direction.

- Fixation of the clavicle to the coracoid is planned. Two 1.6-mm drill holes are made in the anteroposterior center of the clavicle directly over the coracoid; these are spaced approximately 1 cm apart in the medial to lateral direction. A No. 2 nonabsorbable suture is then passed around the coracoid with a semicircular suture passer (coracoid passer). The medial limb is passed through the medial drill hole and the lateral limb is passed through the lateral drill hole.

- Two drill holes are made in the remaining distal clavicle approximately 2 cm from the superior distal edge. These should be placed as far apart in the anterior-posterior plane while still maintaining an adequate bony bridge in all directions.

- Two drill holes are placed in the acromial wafer; adequate distance from the edges of the wafer must be maintained to ensure a sufficient bony bridge.

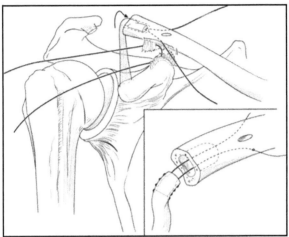

Figure 10-3. Diagram of Weaver-Dunn technique done without an acromial wafer. (From Mazzocca AD, Santangelo SA, Johnson ST, Rios CG, Dumonski ML, Arciero RA. *Am J Sports Med,* 34[2], pp 236-246, copyright © 2006 by SAGE Publications. Reprinted by permission of SAGE Publications.)

- A No. 2 nonabsorbable suture is passed through the CA ligament and through the drill holes in the acromial wafer. The limbs of the suture are passed through the drill holes in the distal clavicle.
- The acromion is reduced to the clavicle by imparting a superiorly directed force through the humerus. Following reduction of the acromion, the sutures from the coracoid to the clavicle are tied. The sutures from the acromial wafer to the distal clavicle then are tied.
- The deltoid is repaired meticulously to the anterior border of the acromion and clavicle. The superficial tissues and skin are repaired according to surgeon preference (Figure 10-3).

Anatomic Coracoclavicular Ligament Reconstruction With Autograft or Allograft

- General anesthesia is induced. The patient is placed into the beach chair position. The operative upper extremity is prepared and draped sterilely.

- An incision along the clavicle is made extending from the distal end medially for 3.5 cm. The medial aspect of the incision is curved slightly anteriorly to aid in exposure of the coracoid. Skin flaps are then developed anteriorly and posteriorly exposing the clavicle.

- A semitendinosus, gracilis, or tibialis allograft or autograft is obtained and cleaned. The graft should be 12 to 14 cm in length and, when folded upon itself, should pass though a 4.5- to 5.5-mm sizing block. Each end of the graft should be secured using a whipstitch technique approximately 3 cm from the center of the graft.

- The base of the coracoid is exposed and a 2.4-mm pin is placed in the coronal center of the base. A reamer of appropriate diameter is introduced over the guide pin. This diameter should allow for the size of the graft when doubled.

- The center of the selected graft is secured using an interference fixation method into the predrilled coracoid, leaving the 2 end limbs free for reconstruction of the conoid and trapezoid ligaments.

- Alternatively, the graft can be looped around the coracoid base; this eliminates using the interference technique, and thereby minimizes the risk of a coracoid fracture. A semicircular passer is passed from medial to lateral around the base of the coracoid. A stout traction suture is then advanced through the passer and the passer is gently removed leaving the suture looped around the base of the coracoid. One limb of the prepared graft can then be secured to the end of the traction suture, and the traction suture is then pulled, advancing the graft around the coracoid, stopping when there are equal lengths of graft on either side of the coracoid.

- One centimeter of distal clavicle can be resected to remove degenerative changes, facilitate reduction of the clavicle to the acromion, and prevent possible future symptomatic degeneration of the AC joint that might occur.

- The positions of the clavicular bone tunnels for placement of the graft limbs are then determined. A 2.4-mm guide pin for the conoid is placed roughly 4.5 cm from the end of the nascent distal clavicle. The bone tunnel should be placed posteriorly to recreate the original insertion of the conoid ligament. An additional 2.4-mm pin is placed approximately 1.5 cm medial to the first pin in the center portion of the clavicle, approximating the original insertion of the trapezoid ligament. These pins are used as guides for a 6- or 7-mm reamer; care is taken not to breach the posterior cortex during tunnel placement for the conoid limb.

- The conoid reconstruction limb is passed through the posteriorly and medially placed hole, and the trapezoid limb is placed through the centrally and laterally placed hole.

- The humerus is loaded in a superior direction, reducing the acromion to the clavicle, and any excess graft is pulled superiorly through the clavicle. The grafts are secured with an interference screw.

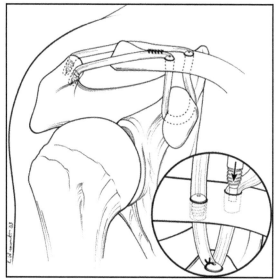

Figure 10-4. Anatomic coracoclavicular reconstruction diagram. (From Mazzocca AD, Arciero RA, Bicos J. *Am J Sports Med*, 35[2], pp 316-329, copyright © 2007 by SAGE Publications. Reprinted by permission of SAGE Publications.)

- Enough excess graft is left to be oversewn with nonabsorbable suture; the remainder is excised. Alternatively, the remaining graft can be secured to the medial acromion crossing the AC joint for further stabilization.
- A meticulous closure of the deltotrapezial fascia is completed using an interlocking stitch and a nonabsorbable suture material. The skin is closed according to surgeon preference (Figures 10-4 and 10-5).

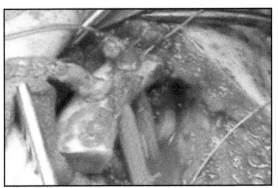

Figure 10-5. Intraoperative anatomic coracoclavicular reconstruction.

Arthroscopic Anatomic Coracoclavicular Reconstruction With Autograft or Allograft

- General anesthesia is induced. The patient is placed into the beach chair position. The operative upper extremity is prepared and draped sterilely.
- The bony landmarks are outlined, as are the anticipated locations of the graft tunnels 4.5 and 3 cm medial to the distal clavicle.
- The standard posterior portal is made and the glenohumeral joint is inspected for any associated pathology. The arthroscope is redirected into the subacromial space through the same skin incision (also see Chapter 12, Figure 12-3).
- An anterolateral portal is localized using a spinal needle. Access to the coracoid process and the AC joint must be ensured using the spinal needle prior to creating the portal.

- A subacromial bursectomy is completed to allow adequate visualization of the subacromial space. The CA ligament is identified and followed to its origin using electrocautery or a shaver to locate the coracoid.
- An anterior portal is localized using a spinal needle to assess access to the superior and inferior aspects of the coracoid. The skin incision for this portal is at the inferomedial quarter of the coracoid; the proximity of the major neurovascular structures must be recognized. A working cannula is introduced into this portal to enable safe access.
- Electrocautery is introduced through the anterior portal and is used to clear the superior and inferior aspects of the "elbow" of the coracoid; the medial and lateral soft-tissue attachments are maintained.
- The AC joint and distal clavicle are débrided, and the distal clavicle is resected to allow impingement-free reduction of the distal clavicle to the acromion.
- An incision is made along the clavicle between the marked locations of the graft tunnels.
- The locations of the tunnels for the limbs of graft reconstruction are localized by placing Kirschner wires through the incision while visualizing the clavicle from the undersurface via the anterolateral portal. The wires are directed toward the coracoid process.
- A cannulated 6-mm reamer is introduced over the wires previously placed into the clavicle at the locations of the insertions of the trapezoid and conoid ligaments. The clavicle is then bicortically reamed over the previously placed Kirschner wires.
- A passing suture is introduced through the anterior portal and passed from lateral to medial inferior to the coracoid, and subsequently through the

reamed posteromedial clavicular tunnel. A second passing suture is introduced and placed over the acromion and through the lateral trapezoid tunnel.

- The medial suture is used to pass the graft around the coracoid and through the medial tunnel. The lateral suture is used to retrieve the other limb of the graft through the lateral tunnel.
- The humerus is loaded in a superior direction, reducing the acromion to the clavicle, and any excess graft is pulled superiorly through the clavicle. The grafts are secured with an interference screw.
- Enough graft is left to be oversewn using nonabsorbable sutures; the remainder is excised.
- The wounds are closed according to surgeon preference.

REHABILITATION

Rehabilitation programs should be defined individually for each patient, taking into account the severity of injury and operation as well as need and demand of the patient. The following suggestions for each procedure can be used as a basic guideline and should be modified according to the progress of the patient.

Distal Clavicle Excision/Resection[2]

- Immobilization for 1 to 3 days followed by a range of motion program.
- Week 1: Passive range of motion—Full external rotation (ER) and internal rotation (IR); forward elevation (FE), scaption, and abduction limited to 90 degrees.
- Week 2: Active assisted range of motion—Full ER and IR; FE, scaption, and abduction limited to 90 degrees. Light isometrics: ER, IR, and triceps.

- Week 3: Active range of motion if tolerated—Full ER and IR; FE, scaption, and abduction limited to 90 degrees.
- Week 4 to 6: Strengthening and active range of motion in all dimensions of shoulder movement. Emphasis should be on scapular stabilizers, since they decrease load to AC joint by maximally retracting the scapula.
- Heavy weight training at 3 months (athletes might need 6 to 12 months to regain peak strength).

Modified Weaver-Dunn Procedure (Coracoacromial Ligament Transfer)[4]

- Immobilization of shoulder for 4 weeks.
- Week 5: Pendulums and passive range of motion—Full ER and IR; FE, scaption, and abduction limited to 90 degrees.
- Week 6: Active assisted and active range of motion—Full ER and IR; FE, scaption, and abduction limited to 90 degrees.
- Weeks 10 to 12: Strengthening and full active range of motion in all dimension of shoulder movement as well as scapula stabilizers.
- Return to sports approximately 4 months after surgery, depending on progress of rehabilitation.

Anatomic Coracoclavicular Ligament Reconstruction With Autograft or Allograft[2]

- Immobilization of shoulder for 4 weeks.
- Week 2: Gentle passive range of motion in supine position—Full ER and IR; FE, scaption, and abduction limited to 90 degrees.
- Weeks 4 to 6: Active range of motion after an acute repair; should be delayed to 6 to 12 weeks after

a chronic repair to allow further healing. In both cases full ER and IR as well as FE, scaption, and abduction limited to 90 degrees are allowed.

- Weeks 6 to 12: Full active range of motion and begin strengthening after acute repair; it should be delayed appropriately (approximately 12 weeks after surgery) after a chronic repair. All dimensions of shoulder movement as well as scapula stabilizers should be considered.
- Heavy weight training can start 3 to 4.5 months after acute repair, but peak strengths might not be reached until 9 to 12 months postoperatively.

OUTCOMES

Acromioclavicular Arthrosis

Surgical Versus Nonsurgical Treatment

There have been no comparisons of surgical and nonsurgical management of AC arthrosis. A course of nonoperative management is the standard of care for treatment of AC arthrosis. In a retrospective review,[1] 93% of patients reported functional improvement and pain relief after corticosteroid injection (for a mean duration of 21 days), but 67% of these patients ultimately underwent distal clavicle excision at a mean of 4 months following injection (level 4 evidence).

Arthroscopic Versus Open Distal Clavicle Excision

In 2007, a randomized, controlled trial limited by a small patient population compared outcomes of surgery after 6 months of conservative treatment.[8] Patients improved following arthroscopic and open distal clavicle excision; although no significant difference was reported, a trend toward more improvement in subjective symptoms (ie, pain) and functional outcomes (ie, return to activities) was noted in the patients treated arthroscopically.

Acromioclavicular Joint Dislocation

Nonoperative Management

The occurrence of degenerative arthrosis of this joint following injury is reported to occur in 50% of patients.[9] Management of this is similar to that of idiopathic degenerative arthrosis of the AC joint.

Operative Management

The modified Weaver-Dunn technique has been the mainstay of treatment of higher grade injuries of the AC joint for years. Many recent publications, however, suggest the anatomic CC reconstruction to result in superior clinical outcomes and biomechanical function.[6,10-12] The optimal technique for anatomic reconstruction continues to evolve as advances are made with innovative techniques and materials. Maintaining the length of the clavicle in an acute injury has been suggested to improve the stability of the reconstruction.[6]

POTENTIAL COMPLICATIONS

Open/Arthroscopic Distal Clavicle Excision

- Instability is the major complication of this procedure. Excessive resection of the distal clavicle (greater than 0.5 to 1 cm) and failure to repair the AC capsule and deltopectoral fascia can lead to cephalad/caudad and anteroposterior instability, respectively.
- Failure to resect an adequate amount of distal clavicle can result in failure to relieve symptoms.
- Deltoid dehiscence due to inadequate repair following an open resection can cause significant disability in the shoulder.

Modified Weaver-Dunn Procedure/ Coracoclavicular Reconstruction

- Failure of the reconstruction and subsequent recurrent instability
- Infection
- Injury to neurovascular structures medial to coracoid during procedure
- Tunnel expansion has been reported in the anatomic CC reconstruction; the clinical significance of this is unknown[13]

REFERENCES

1. Jacobs AK, Sallay PI. Therapeutic efficacy of corticosteroid injections in the acromioclavicular joint. *Biomed Sci Instrum.* 1997;34:380-385.
2. Mazzocca AD, Arciero RA, Bicos J. Evaluation and treatment of acromioclavicular joint injuries. *Am J Sports Med.* 2007;35(2):316-329.
3. Weaver J, Dunn H. Treatment of acromioclavicular injuries, especially complete acromioclavicular separation. *J Bone Joint Surg Am.* 1972;54:1187-1194.
4. Millett PJ, Braun S, Gobezie R, Pacheco IH. Acromioclavicular joint reconstruction with coracoacromial ligament transfer using the docking technique. *BMC Musculoskelet Disord.* 2009;10:6.
5. Lee SJ, Nicholas SJ, Akizuki KH, McHugh MP, Kremenic IJ, Ben-Avi S. Reconstruction of the coracoclavicular ligaments with tendon grafts: a comparative biomechanical study. *Am J Sports Med.* 2003;31:648-655.
6. Mazzocca A, Santangelo S, Johnson S, Rios C, Dumonski M, Arciero R. A biomechanical evaluation of an anatomical coracoclavicular ligament reconstruction. *Am J Sports Med.* 2006;34:236-246.
7. Costic RS, Labriola JE, Rodosky MW, Debski RE. Biomechanical rationale for development of anatomical reconstruction of coracoclavicular ligaments after complete acromioclavicular joint dislocations. *Am J Sports Med.* 2004;32:1929-1936.

8. Freedman BA, Javernick MA, O'Brien FP, Ross AE, Doukas WC. Arthroscopic versus open distal clavicle excision: comparative results at six months and one year from a randomized, prospective clinical trial. *J Shoulder Elbow Surg.* 2007;16(4):413-418.

9. Bergfeld JA, Andrish JT, Clancy WG. Evaluation of the acromioclavicular joint following first- and second-degree sprains. *Am J Sports Med.* 1978;6(4):153-159.

10. Tauber M, Gordon K, Koller H, Fox M, Resch H. Semitendinosus tendon graft versus a modified Weaver-Dunn procedure for acromioclavicular joint reconstruction in chronic cases: a prospective comparative study. *Am J Sports Med.* 2009;37:181-190.

11. Harris RI, Wallace AL, Harper GD, Goldberg JA, Sonnabend DH, Walsh WR. Structural properties of the intact and reconstructed coracoclavicular ligament complex. *Am J Sport Med.* 2000;28:103-108.

12. Jari R, Constic RS, Rodosky MW, Debski RE. Biomechanical function of surgical procedures for acromioclavicular joint dislocations. *Arthroscopy.* 2004;20:237-245.

13. Yoo JC, Choi NH, Kim SY, Lim TK. Distal clavicle tunnel widening after coracoclavicular ligament reconstruction with semitendinosus tendon: a case report. *J Shoulder Elbow Surg.* 2006;15:256-259.

Relevant Review Articles

Shaffer BS. Painful conditions of the acromioclavicular joint. *J Am Acad Orthop Surg.* 1999;7(3):176-188.

Simovitch R, Sanders B, Ozbaydar M, Lavery K, Warner JJP. Acromioclavicular joint injuries: diagnosis and management. *J Am Acad Orthop Surg.* 2009;17(4):207-219.

CHAPTER 11

IMPINGEMENT AND PARTIAL-THICKNESS ROTATOR CUFF TEARS

Sepp Braun, MD; Florian Elser, MD; and Peter J. Millett, MD, MSc

MECHANISM OF INJURY/ PATHOPHYSIOLOGY

The subacromial space presents with various pathologies that range from rotator cuff tendinitis and impingement syndrome to partial- and full-thickness rotator cuff tears (PTRCTs and FTRCTs, respectively). Several types of impingement have been described in the literature, which include "classic" subacromial impingement, secondary impingement, and internal impingement.

Recognition and treatment of impingement is important not only for symptomatic relief, but because impingement ultimately can lead to PTRCT. Most commonly located on the articular side of the supraspinatus tendon, PTRCTs occur increasingly with age.[1] Although some partial tears may heal without surgical intervention, most tears appear to enlarge over time if treated nonoperatively.[2] PTRCTs in overhead-throwing athletes are common and often present with symptoms different from the general population. Tears are located more anteriorly and posteriorly and require different treatment strategies due to the needs of overhead sports.

Rohde RS, Millett PJ, eds.
Evaluation and Management of Common Upper Extremity Disorders: A Practical Handbook (pp 185-206).
© 2011 Taylor & Francis Group.

Causes of Impingement

- **"Classic" impingement** (outlet or external impingement)[3,4] results from compression of the rotator cuff between the coracoacromial (CA) arch and the humeral head. Anatomical variants such as a hooked acromion, acromioclavicular (AC) joint arthritis with osteophyte formation, and a laterally sloping acromion have been proposed as predisposing factors.
- **Secondary impingement** (nonoutlet) describes a dynamic process; the subacromial arch is normal, but the humeral head and rotator cuff are strained superiorly. Commonly seen in athletes with capsular contracture, this results when forward elevation of the arm causes obligate anterosuperior translation of the humeral head.[5] Posterior capsular tightness creates vector imbalance resulting in migration of the humeral head with secondary rotator cuff symptoms.[6]
- **Internal impingement** occurs when the undersurface of the rotator cuff contacts the posterior-superior labrum when the arm is held in maximum external rotation and abduction.[7] This can result in superior labrum anterior-posterior (SLAP) lesions, PTRCTs, hyperlaxity of the anterior glenohumeral ligaments, and posterior capsular contractures. Internal impingement most likely is caused by shoulder girdle muscle fatigue resulting from a lack of conditioning or overthrowing.[8-11]

Causes of Partial-Thickness Rotator Cuff Tears

- **Intrinsic** causes related to the aging process affect the vascularity, metabolism, and tensile strength of tendons, resulting in tendinopathy. This typically is associated with articular-side tears and delamination.

- **Extrinsic** causes usually relate to impingement by CA arch abnormalities. This typically is associated with bursal-side tears, but some theorize that this also causes articular-side tears.[12]
- **Traumatic** injuries most often are associated with articular-side tears.[13]

Causes of Partial-Thickness Rotator Cuff Tears in Overhead-Throwing Athletes

- Large eccentric traction forces on the supraspinatus and infraspinatus tendons during the throwing motion can cause PTRCT.[14]
- Minor instability and fatigue of the dynamic stabilizers cause anterior subluxation, which in turn causes secondary impingement of the rotator cuff on the posterior edge of the glenoid and repetitive microtrauma to the rotator cuff.[15]
- Posterosuperior subluxation of the humerus from posterior capsule contracture and repetitive torsional and shear overload generated by hyperexternal rotation causes these tears, given the association with posterior type 2 SLAP tears.[16]

Classification

In general, classification of PTRCTs depends upon the location (which tendon and which surface), depth, and cause of the tear. A more detailed classification scheme to include location of tear (bursal, articular, or intratendinous) and its depth (grade 1: <1/3, grade 2: 1/3, grade 3: >1/2 of the cuff thickness) has been described (Figure 11-1).[17]

PTRCTs are most commonly located on the articular side in the supraspinatus tendon. Less frequently, partial

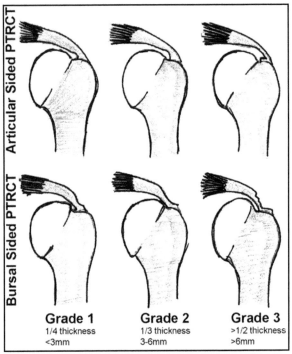

Figure 11-1. Classification of partial-thickness rotator cuff tears.

tears occur on the bursal side or intratendinous in the infraspinatus, subscapularis, and teres minor tendons.

KEY HISTORY POINTS

- Subdeltoid pain frequently is described as radiating down the arm and the brachium.

- Pain frequently is worse at night and often keeps the patient awake.
- Primary impingement rarely is seen in patients less than 40 years old. Instability of the glenohumeral joint, lesions of the rotator interval, or SLAP lesions can mimic impingement syndromes in younger patients.
- Patients describe weakness of the arm, especially in cases of PTRCT.
- PTRCTs sometimes generate more pain than FTRCTs.[18]

KEY EXAMINATION POINTS

- As for all shoulder pathologies, a complete physical examination including inspection for muscle atrophy, skin color, and warmth is suggested, as well as documentation of the passive and active range of motion.
- In the case of isolated impingement, range of motion usually is not limited, but active abduction and internal rotation behind the back are painful.
- PTRCT may result in restricted internal rotation from posterior capsular tightness and glenohumeral joint contracture.[19]
- Passive motion of the arm is most painful through the arc of 60 to 120 degrees of abduction.[13]
- Active lowering of the arm following passive elevation can elicit pain.
- An apparent loss of strength or decrease in active range of motion can be caused by pain inhibition in cases of impingement and PTRCT.
- Clinical tests for all rotator cuff muscles are negative for patients with isolated impingement syndrome, but may be positive for those with PTRCT (for further descriptions, see Appendix).

- ☐ Supraspinatus muscle
  - Starter test: Strength of abduction in neutral arm position
  - Jobe test: Upward strength of the abducted and 30 forward flexed arm
- ☐ Subscapularis muscle
  - Strength of internal rotation
  - Lift-off test
  - Belly press test
- ☐ Infraspinatus muscle
  - Strength of external rotation
  - External rotation lag sign
- The following primary and secondary impingement tests are positive:
  - ☐ Hawkins-Kennedy impingement test
  - ☐ Neer impingement test
  - ☐ Jobe test
- Examination for instability (see Chapter 14) is essential for a correct diagnosis.
- Positive SLAP tests can indicate subtle instability that also can lead to impingement-like symptoms.
- Presence of positive lag signs can distinguish FTRCTs from PTRCTs, which would present without lag signs. In contrast, impingement tests are frequently positive in patients with PTRCT, but not necessarily in FTRCT.
- The following additional clinical tests are recommended for overhead-throwing athletes:
  - ☐ Examination of the shoulder's anterior-posterior and inferior stability (see Chapter 14)
  - ☐ Glenohumeral internal rotation deficit test: Increased external rotation in abduction on the patient's dominant side with concomitant loss of internal rotation can cause internal impingement

Because of its nonspecific nature, PTRCT can be difficult to diagnose clinically; symptoms are similar to and

overlap with those of subacromial bursitis, bicipital tendinitis, and mild cases of frozen shoulder. It is important
to keep in mind that PTRCT often can be associated with
the following shoulder lesions:

- Biceps tendon fraying or rupture[20,21]
- Labral degeneration or tearing (up to one-third of
  patients)[20,22]
- Posterosuperior labral lesions or osteochondral
  lesions of the humeral head sometimes present in
  throwing athletes[23]

ADDITIONAL TESTING OR IMAGING

- Radiographs
  - □ True anterior-posterior view
  - □ Scapular outlet view (scapulolateral view with
    center beam directed 10 degrees caudally
    demonstrates acromion morphology)
  - □ Axillary lateral view shows os acromiale,
    which can cause impingement symptoms
  - □ Impingement radiograph (anterior-posterior
    view with 30 degrees downward tilt can dem-
    onstrate anteroinferior acromial spurs)
  - □ Apical oblique (Garth) or West Point axillary
    view if glenohumeral instability is suspected
- Patients respond well to the **local anesthetic injection test** in the subacromial space. The injection is
  administered at the same starting point and direction as the arthroscope is introduced into the subacromial space from the standard posterior portal.
- **Ultrasound** by an experienced provider is highly
  sensitive for PTRCT.[24]
- **Magnetic resonance imaging** (MRI) can demonstrate the presence of subacromial bursitis or rotator
  cuff tears, although it is less reliable for detecting
  PTRCT than FTRCT. Capsular structures can be assessed, as can the long head of the biceps tendon
  complex.

- T1-weighted imaging of PTRCT demonstrates increased signal in the rotator cuff without evidence of tendon discontinuity.
- T2-weighted imaging of PTRCT shows increased signal with an intratendinous focal defect or a focal defect limited to one surface of the tendon.
- Concomitant use of arthrography can improve detection of rotator cuff pathology, especially in PTRCT.[25]
- Sequences obtained using special patient positioning, such as abducted-externally rotated views, improve visualization of the rotator cuff and posterior-superior labrum in throwing athletes.[25]
- Diagnosis-specific sequencing such as fat suppression, spin-echo and proton-density techniques, and higher-power magnets (3.0 T) allow for an unprecedented level of soft-tissue detail.[25]

TREATMENT OPTIONS: NONOPERATIVE

- Physical therapy can be initiated for rotator cuff strengthening and recentering of the humeral head in the glenoid socket.
- Stretching of the joint capsule can be attempted using the sleeper stretch (flexion and internal rotation to address posterior capsular contracture) and/or cross-arm stretch (horizontal adduction exercises to stretch posterior capsule).
- Modification of daily recreational and work activities can be initiated.
- Nonsteroidal anti-inflammatory medications and/or local corticosteroid injection can decrease subacromial bursal inflammation.

TREATMENT OPTIONS: OPERATIVE

Patients whose symptoms are refractory to 6 months of nonoperative treatment generally are considered for surgery. A patient's activity level, individual needs, and mechanical pathomechanisms (eg, spurs) may shorten this time period.

For patients with PTRCTs due to extrinsic outlet impingement, intrinsic tendinopathy, or instability, nonoperative treatment similar to that recommended for impingement syndrome is possible. As described previously, most tears appear to enlarge over time if treated nonoperatively.

Operative Treatment Options

- Capsular release to address capsular contractures that are not responding to stretching programs
- Subacromial decompression (acromioplasty) to resect spurs on the undersurface of the acromion
- Tear débridement
- Tear débridement and acromioplasty
- Rotator cuff repair and acromioplasty
- Additional healing response and bone marrow stimulation can be incited by perforating the cortex of the bone in the area of the rotator cuff footprint; bone marrow-derived stem cells can stimulate healing of the tendon

SURGICAL ANATOMY

Landmarks for Arthroscopic Approach

- AC joint
- Coracoid process
- Anterolateral and posterolateral corner of the acromion

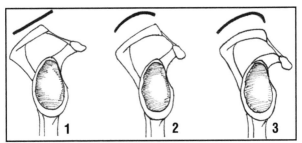

Figure 11-2. Bigliani classification of acromion types.

Portals

- Standard posterior viewing portal
- Anterior-superior and lateral working portal
- Additional lateral portals as needed

The Subacromial Space[26]

- The subacromial space is confined superiorly by the acromion, the CA ligament, and the coracoid process.
- The subacromial and subdeltoid bursa are found in the subacromial space.
- The rotator cuff is found at the floor of the subacromial space.
- The "fornix humeri," built by the acromion, the CA ligament, and the coracoid process, is the roof of the subacromial space. The CA arch is 39% larger than the radius of the humeral head.[27,28]
- Acromion types (Figure 11-2)[29]
    - ☐ Flat (Bigliani type 1)
    - ☐ Curved (Bigliani type 2)
    - ☐ Hooked (Bigliani type 3)
- Rotator cuff anatomy

The vascularity on the articular surface of the rotator cuff is relatively low compared with the bursal side. There is a critical zone of hypovascularity near the insertion of the supraspinatus tendon on the humerus.[30,31] Further, compared to the thick, parallel collagen bundles found near the surface of the bursal side of the rotator cuff, the bundles on the articular side are thinner and less uniform. The bursal side can withstand greater deformation and has greater tensile strength than the articular side.[32] This might account for the greater frequency of articular side tears.

PROCEDURES

Subacromial Decompression/ Acromioplasty

- Patient in general anesthesia; interscalene nerve block may improve patient's postoperative comfort.
- Beach chair positioning on a shoulder operating table, standard draping, and use of a pneumatic arm holder are very helpful.
- The arthroscope is introduced into the subacromial space through the standard posterior portal.
- The CA ligament and the anterior border of the acromion are palpated with the tip of the trocar.
- The CA ligament preserves the CA arch (fornix humeri) and is **not** resected.
- A second portal is placed anteriorly at the lateral border of the acromion, perpendicular to the arthroscope.
- A débrider is introduced to perform the **bursectomy**; visualization of the rotator cuff, the undersurface of the acromion, and the AC joint is maintained.
- Tissue medial to the AC joint is well vascularized; débridement of this is avoided to prevent bleeding.

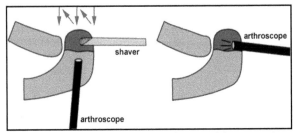

Figure 11-3. Steps of an arthroscopic subacromial decompression.

Acromioplasty should be limited to a conversion of the acromion to a flat type 1.

- □ Resection of spurs and osteophytes with a burr is critical.
- □ The anterolateral border of the acromion is identified; this is helped by use of radio frequency ablation. The AC ligament is located first by palpating the bone and soft tissue, and the soft tissue is débrided until the bone is visualized easily. Some authors perform a partial release of the anterolateral portion of the CA ligament.
- □ The anterior part of the acromion is resected, starting anterior and lateral with the burr inserted through the lateral portal (Figure 11-3).
- □ Particularly in patients with a curved type 2 acromion, there is a significant danger of resecting too much bone. The resection line should be oriented on the undersurface of the anterior third of the acromion.
- □ Co-planing of the lateral clavicle is performed if necessary.

Arthroscopic Repair of Partial-Thickness Rotator Cuff Tears

- Advantages of an arthroscopic repair include visualization of the articular surface of the cuff, no need for detachment of the deltoid muscle, and the ability to examine the shoulder completely for intra- and extra-articular co-pathologies.
    - □ Visualization (beach chair position)
        - Patient in general anesthesia; interscalene nerve block may improve patient's postoperative comfort.
        - Beach chair positioning on a shoulder operating table, standard draping, and use of a pneumatic arm holder are very helpful.
        - The undersurface of the rotator cuff is visualized with the arthroscope in the standard posterior portal and rotated to view laterally; the shoulder is abducted 30 degrees, externally rotated 30 to 45 degrees, and flexed slightly forward.[33]
        - The arthroscope can be swept along the insertion of the rotator cuff on the proximal humerus to visualize the biceps, supraspinatus, infraspinatus, and teres minor attachment sites.
        - Internal impingement lesions are best viewed with the shoulder abducted 90 degrees and the arm held in maximum external rotation.
    - □ Articular tears sometimes require gentle débridement for visualization of the undersurface; integrity of the rotator cuff can be assessed using a probe inserted through the anterior portal.

□ Bursal tears can be obscured by hypertrophic bursitis; débridement of this improves visualization. Subacromial spurring or a prominent CA ligament—"impingement lesions"—might be identifiable in readily visible tears. Full examination of the bursal surface is accomplished using both the posterior and lateral portals for viewing while putting the shoulder through full range of motion. The supraspinatus insertion is examined by rotating the shoulder internally and externally while the shoulder is slightly abducted.

□ The rotator cuff should be visualized completely through the lateral and/or anterior subacromial portal; careful inspection of tendons is necessary as FTRCTs can be present.

□ Intratendinous tears cannot be identified during arthroscopic surgery; these are diagnosed by history, physical examination, and MRI findings only.

Open Surgical Repair

- Advantages include good visualization of the bursal side of the cuff and the ability to palpate tendons for intratendinous tears.
- Disadvantages include difficulty visualizing the articular side of the cuff, inability to identify concomitant shoulder pathology, and relative invasiveness with potential related damage.

Mini-Open Technique

- Combines arthroscopic examination of glenohumeral joint and subacromial decompression with mini-open repair of PTRCT if needed.
- Mini-open repair uses a deltoid-splitting technique. Care should be taken to avoid going too

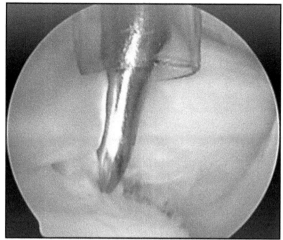

Figure 11-4. Healing response for partial-thickness rotator cuff tear with microfracture awl.

far anteriorly, which can jeopardize the deltoid's attachment to the acromion.

Treatment Recommendations

Bursal-Surface Tears

- Débridement if tear is greater than 50% of tendon thickness; consider healing response and bone marrow stimulation (Figure 11-4)
- Repair if tear is greater than 50% of tendon thickness[34]
- Acromioplasty or subacromial decompression without acromioplasty if there is hypertrophic bursal tissue and flat acromial morphology

Articular-Surface Tears (Partial Articular-Sided Supraspinatus Tendon Avulsion)

- Examine carefully for evidence of instability and address if necessary (see Chapter 14).
- Acromioplasty in the older patient with a degenerative articular-surface tear; consider healing response/bone marrow stimulation.
- Repair in younger patients if tear is greater than 50% of tendon thickness.[34]
  - Complete partial tear to full-thickness tear and repair.
  - Partial articular-sided supraspinatus tendon avulsion repair: Introduce anchor and perforate tendon with the anchor for repair.[35,36]
- Healing response/bone marrow stimulation in younger patients with tears greater than 50% of tendon thickness.

REHABILITATION

Subacromial Decompression/ Acromioplasty

- A regular arm sling is used for comfort only for up to 2 weeks; early full range of motion is encouraged.
- Physical therapy without limits for passive and active range of motion is initiated, and strengthening exercises begin 3 to 4 weeks postoperatively as tolerated.

Repair of Partial-Thickness Rotator Cuff Tears

- An abduction sling is used for 4 weeks.
- Free passive range of motion and active assisted abduction are allowed for 2 weeks.

- Full active range of motion begins on week 3.
- Overhead activity and lifting more than 5 pounds generally begins after 6 weeks, with advanced resistance strengthening and proprioception training starting at 8 weeks postoperatively.

OUTCOMES

Arthroscopic management of subacromial impingement with acromioplasty has a 70% to 90% success rate.[37] This is particularly true for extrinsic or outlet impingement syndromes, most commonly caused by degenerative acromion spurs or osteophytes at the AC joint. This procedure is **not** successful in cases of internal impingement or if the humeral head is decentered by capsular contractures or instability.

Results of Operative Procedures

Tear débridement alone allows for assessment of the tear but also can relieve mechanical irritation[38] and remove inflammatory cells[38]; this has resulted in 50% to 94% satisfactory results.[14,22,39]

- Arthroscopic subacromial decompression for treatment of PTRCTs is associated with 75% to 83% satisfactory results[39-41]; this is particularly successful when used to treat bursal-side tears.[20]
- Open treatment of PTRCT by performing complete excision of damaged tissue followed by open repair is reported to have over 80% satisfactory results.[42]

POTENTIAL COMPLICATIONS

- **Misdiagnosis:** Accurate diagnosis of impingement syndromes is necessary to avoid surgical failures. Several other shoulder pathologies, including glenohumeral instability, early adhesive capsulitis, and AC joint degeneration, all can mimic and/or coexist with true impingement.

- **Inappropriate resection:** Resecting too little or too much bone from the acromion can lead to failure of the procedure. Unfortunately, the latter is hard to address with revision surgery. To avoid excessive decompression, the preoperative radiographs must be evaluated carefully and the patient's individual anatomy appreciated while planning the surgical procedure. When the acromion is curved, decompression with the burr solely using the posterior portal can result in a complete anterior acromionectomy; to avoid this, we recommend intermittent instrument changes between anterolateral and posterior portals.
- **Progression of tear:** PTRCT can progress to FTRCT even if treated operatively.
- Postoperative stiffness and wound infection are general risks of shoulder surgery.

REFERENCES

1. Sher JS, Uribe JW, Posada A, Murphy BJ, Zlatkin MB. Abnormal findings on magnetic resonance images of asymptomatic shoulders. *J Bone Joint Surg Am.* 1995;77(1): 10-15.
2. Yamanaka K, Matsumoto T. The joint side tear of the rotator cuff. A followup study by arthrography. *Clin Orthop Relat Res.* 1994;304:68-73.
3. Neer CS 2nd. Impingement lesions. *Clin Orthop Relat Res.* 1983;173:70-77.
4. Neer CS 2nd. Anterior acromioplasty for the chronic impingement syndrome in the shoulder. 1972. *J Bone Joint Surg Am.* 2005;87(6):1399.
5. Sethi PM, Tibone JE, Lee TQ. Quantitative assessment of glenohumeral translation in baseball players: a comparison of pitchers versus nonpitching athletes. *Am J Sports Med.* 2004;32(7):1711-1715.
6. Ticker JB, Biem GM, Warner JJP. Recognition and treatment of refractory posterior capsular contracture of the shoulder. *Arthroscopy.* 2000;16:27-34.

7. Walch G, Boileau P, Noel E, et al. Impingement of the deep surface of the supraspinatus tendon on the postero-superior glenoid rim: an arthroscopic study. *J Shoulder Elbow Surg.* 1992;1:238-245.

8. Jobe CM. Posterior superior glenoid impingement: expanded spectrum. *Arthroscopy.* 1995;11:530-536.

9. Jobe CM. Superior glenoid impingement. *Arthroscopy.* 1997;28:137-143.

10. Paly KJ, Jobe FW, Pink MM, Kvitne RS, El Attrache NS. Arthroscopic findings in the overhand throwing athlete: evidence of posterior internal impingement of the rotator cuff. *Arthroscopy.* 2000;16:35-40.

11. Jobe FW, Kvitne RS, Giangarra CE. Shoulder pain in the throwing athlete. The relationship of anterior instability and rotator cuff impingement. *Orthop Rev.* 1989;18:963-975.

12. Gartsman GM, Milne JC. Articular surface partial-thickness rotator cuff tears. *J Shoulder Elbow Surg.* 1995;4(6): 409-415.

13. Itoi E, Tabata S. Incomplete rotator cuff tears. Results of operative treatment. *Clin Orthop Relat Res.* 1992;284: 128-135.

14. Andrews JR, Broussard TS, Carson WG. Arthroscopy of the shoulder in the management of partial tears of the rotator cuff: a preliminary report. *Arthroscopy.* 1985;1(2): 117-122.

15. Davidson PA, Elattrache NS, Jobe CM, Jobe FW. Rotator cuff and posterior-superior glenoid labrum injury associated with increased glenohumeral motion: a new site of impingement. *J Shoulder Elbow Surg.* 1995;4(5):384-390.

16. Burkhart SS, Morgan CD, Kibler WB. The disabled throwing shoulder: spectrum of pathology Part I: patho-anatomy and biomechanics. *Arthroscopy.* 2003;19(4): 404-420.

17. Ellman H. Diagnosis and treatment of incomplete rotator cuff tears. *Clin Orthop Relat Res.* 1990;254:64-74.

18. Bey MJ, Ramsey ML, Soslowsky LJ. Intratendinous strain fields of the supraspinatus tendon: effect of a surgically created articular-surface rotator cuff tear. *J Shoulder Elbow Surg.* 2002;11(6):562-569.

19. Fukuda H, Craig EV, Yamanaka K, Hamada K. Partial-thickness rotator cuff tears. In: Burkhead WZJ, ed. *Rotator Cuff Disorders.* Vols 174-181. Baltimore, MD: Williams & Wilkins; 1996.

20. Ryu RK. Arthroscopic subacromial decompression: a clinical review. *Arthroscopy.* 1992;8(2):141-147.

21. Paulos LE, Franklin JL. Arthroscopic shoulder decompression development and application. A five year experience. *Am J Sports Med.* 1990;18(3):235-244.

22. Snyder SJ, Pachelli AF, Del Pizzo W, Friedman MJ, Ferkel RD, Pattee G. Partial thickness rotator cuff tears: results of arthroscopic treatment. *Arthroscopy.* 1991;7(1):1-7.

23. Walch G, Boileau P, Noel E, Donell ST. Impingement of the deep surface of the supraspinatus tendon of the posterosuperior glenoid rim: an arthroscopic study. *J Shoulder Elbow Surg.* 1992;1:238-245.

24. Wiener SN, Seitz WH Jr. Sonography of the shoulder in patients with tears of the rotator cuff: accuracy and value for selecting surgical options. *AJR Am J Roentgenol.* 1993;160(1):103-107.

25. Murray PJ, Shaffer BS. Clinical update: MR imaging of the shoulder. *Sports Med Arthrosc.* 2009;17(1):40-48.

26. Neer CS 2nd, Poppen NK. Supraspinatus outlet. *Orthop Trans.* 1987;11:234.

27. Putz R, Liebermann J, Reichelt A. [The function of the coracoacromial ligament]. *Acta Anat (Basel).* 1988;131(2):140-145.

28. Ogawa K, Toyama Y, Ishige S, Matsui K. [Fracture of the coracoid process: its classification and pathomechanism]. *Nippon Seikeigeka Gakkai Zasshi.* 1990;64(10):909-919.

29. Bigliani LU, Morrison D, April DW. The morphology of the acromion and its relationship to rotator cuff tears. *Orthop Trans.* 1986;10:216.

30. Rothman RH, Parke WW. The vascular anatomy of the rotator cuff. *Clin Orthop Relat Res.* 1965;41:176-186.

31. Lohr JF, Uhthoff HK. The microvascular pattern of the supraspinatus tendon. *Clin Orthop Relat Res.* 1990;254:35-38.

32. Nakajima T, Rokuuma N, Hamada K, Tomatsu T, Fukuda H. Histologic and biomechanical characteristics of the supraspinatus tendon: reference to rotator cuff tearing. *J Shoulder Elbow Surg.* 1994;3:79-87.

33. McConville OR, Iannotti JP. Partial-thickness tears of the rotator cuff: evaluation and management. *J Am Acad Orthop Surg.* 1999;7(1):32-43.

34. Weber SC. Arthroscopic debridement and acromioplasty versus mini-open repair in the management of significant partial-thickness tears of the rotator cuff. *Orthop Clin North Am.* 1997;28:79-82.

35. Ide J, Maeda S, Takagi K. Arthroscopic transtendon repair of partial-thickness articular-side tears of the rotator cuff: anatomical and clinical study. *Am J Sports Med.* 2005;33(11):1672-1679.

36. Snyder SJ. Arthroscopic repair of partial articular supraspinatus tendon avulsions: PASTA lesions of the rotator cuff tendon. In: Snyder SJ, ed. *Shoulder Arthroscopy.* Philadelphia, PA: Lippincott Williams and Wilkins; 2003: 219-229.

37. Ellman H. Arthroscopic subacromial decompression: analysis of one- to three-year results. *Arthroscopy.* 1987;3(3):173-181.

38. Wolff AB, Sethi P, Sutton KM, Covey AS, Magit DP. Partial-thickness rotator cuff tears. *J Am Acad Ortho Surg.* 2006;14:715-725.

39. Ogilvie-Harris DJ, Wiley AM. Arthroscopic surgery of the shoulder. A general appraisal. *J Bone Joint Surg Br.* 1986;68(2):201-207.

40. Gartsman GM. Arthroscopic acromioplasty for lesions of the rotator cuff. *J Bone Joint Surg Am.* 1990;72(2): 169-180.

41. Esch JC, Ozerkis LR, Helgager JA, Kane N, Lilliott N. Arthroscopic subacromial decompression: results according to the degree of rotator cuff tear. *Arthroscopy.* 1988;4(4):241-249.

42. Itoi E, Minagawa H, Sato T, Sato K, Tabata S. Isokinetic strength after tears of the supraspinatus tendon. *J Bone Joint Surg Br.* 1997;79(1):77-82.

Relevant Review Articles

Fukuda H. The management of partial-thickness tears of the rotator cuff. *J Bone Joint Surg Br.* 2003;85(1):3-11.

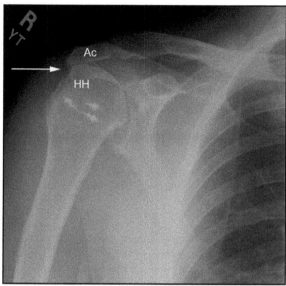

Figure 12-1. Anteroposterior radiograph of the shoulder demonstrating superior migration of the humeral head (HH) with a decreased humeroacromial interval (white arrow) after a previously failed RC repair. Ac=acromion.

- Degenerative changes consistent with RC arthropathy (anteroposterior, axillary)

Computed tomography can visualize bony defects and the addition of arthography allows assessment of RC tears, but it is not the ideal modality for visualization of soft tissues.

The advantages of using **ultrasound** include dynamic testing and low cost. The major disadvantages are that the technique is highly dependent on the skill of the operator and does not evaluate other possible intra-articular sources of shoulder pain including labral tears and biceps tendon pathology.

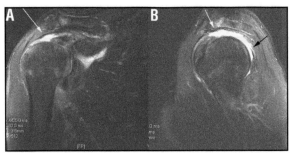

Figure 12-2. (A) T2 weighted coronal MRI image demonstrating a full-thickness tear of the supraspinatus (white arrow). (B) T2 weighted sagittal MRI image demonstrating full-thickness tears of the supraspinatus (white arrow) and infraspinatus (black arrow) tendons.

Magnetic resonance imaging (MRI) and arthrography, although more expensive, have become the standard for evaluating the RC at many centers. These techniques provide a detailed view of the RC tendons, assess other shoulder pathology, and allow for preoperative planning (Figure 12-2). MRI may also demonstrate atrophy and fatty infiltration of the RC.[12]

Direct comparisons of ultrasound, MRI, and MRI with arthrogram have been reported. Ultrasound and MRI have been shown to have a similar sensitivity, specificity, and overall accuracy.[13-15] MRI arthrography is superior to both ultrasound and plain MRI in terms of sensitivity and specificity for visualizing partial- and full-thickness RC tears[13]; the overall accuracy has been reported to be 95% for partial- and 98% for full-thickness tears.[16]

Classification

RC tears are classified as acute, chronic (greater than 3 months), and acute-on-chronic. They also typically are

Table 12-1. Classification for
Full-Thickness Rotator Cuff Tears

Grade/Classification	Greatest Dimension of Tear
I/Small	<1 cm
II/Medium	1 to 3 cm
III/Large	3 to 5 cm
IV/Massive	>5 cm

Data from Cofield RH, Parvizi J, Hoffmeyer PJ, Lanzer WL, Ilstrup DM, Rowland CM. Surgical repair of chronic rotator cuff tears. A prospective long-term study. *J Bone Joint Surg Am.* 2001;83-A(1):71-77.

classified as full or partial thickness and are further stratified by size.

- Full-thickness tears are classified by the size of the tear in largest dimension as small (>1 cm), medium (1 to 3 cm), large (3 to 5 cm), or massive (>5 cm) (Table 12-1).
- Tears also are classified by the number of tendons affected, with more than 2 affected tendons considered indicative of a massive tear.
- Extent of retraction typically is not considered in classification but may be highly important when considering repair. If the tendon retraction would preclude sufficient repair, a tendon transfer may be considered.
- Fatty infiltration and atrophy of the muscles also are noted and can be classified as suggested by Goutallier and colleagues.[12] The extent of fatty degeneration is taken into consideration in determining which tears are reparable.

Treatment Options: Nonoperative

The goal of treatment of RC pathology is to alleviate pain, restore function, and prevent long-term complications including arthrosis. The mainstay of nonoperative treatment is divided into medical treatment (systemic augmented by local modalities) and physical therapy.

- Systemic medical therapy includes acetaminophen for pain relief and/or regular use of nonsteroidal anti-inflammatory drugs (NSAIDs).
- Local medical therapy includes injections of corticosteroids with or without local anesthetic into the subacromial bursa. Injections typically are reserved for patients with continued pain after failing other nonoperative modalities; the authors may administer injections every 3 to 6 months for a total not to exceed 3 injections, as multiple injections may increase the risk of tendon rupture. Results are highly dependent on the accuracy of injection, and ultrasound guidance may be of benefit.[17-19]
- Physical therapy entails a series of exercises initially aimed at pain control, progressing to range of motion, and finally focusing on strengthening to prevent stiffness and restore strength and function.
  - Adjuvant therapies such as therapeutic ultrasound, extracorporeal shock wave therapy, laser therapy, and iontophoresis have not shown any significant efficacy in the treatment of RC pathology.

Treatment Options: Operative

The indications for operative intervention for RC disease are based on characteristics of the pathology, response to nonoperative modalities, and patient goals. Surgery is recommended more frequently in recent years secondary to advances in minimally invasive arthroscopic techniques. However, in the literature, indications rarely are reported, leaving no clear consensus on when to operate.[20] Common indications include the following:

- Impingement and partial-thickness tears with persistent or moderate pain at rest and/or with function after an initial trial (3 to 6 months) of conservative treatment (see Chapter 11)
- An acute full-thickness tear in a young patient (less than 60 years), as delayed repair may be more difficult
- Full-thickness tears in older patients after failure of nonoperative treatment or in a higher demand patient
- Massive tears in older patients involving loss of function and continued pain with good muscle quality on MRI
- **Surgical management** may involve subacromial decompression, acromioplasty, débridement, and/or anatomic repair of the RC. Operative repair has evolved significantly over the past decade from formal open and mini-open techniques to double-row, anatomic arthroscopic fixation.
  - □ Open RC repair involves complete detachment of the deltoid from the acromion to expose the tendons; the axillary nerve is at risk distally.
  - □ Mini-open RC repair uses a deltoid-splitting approach (without detachment of the deltoid); the axillary nerve may be injured if deltoid split is too distal.
  - □ Arthroscopic repair is considered minimally invasive, typically utilizes 4 portals (as detailed in the Procedures section), and allows management of the majority of tears, although certain patterns may require an open approach.

- In patients with irreparable massive tears, tendon transfers and reverse total shoulder arthroplasty should be considered. The latissimus dorsi and/or teres major tendon may be transferred to the greater tuberosity for the patient with a deficient posterior cuff (an intact subscapularis is essential), while the pectoralis major may be transferred to the lesser tuberosity for an irreparable subscapularis tear.

SURGICAL ANATOMY

- The RC is composed of the supraspinatus, infraspinatus, teres minor, and subscapularis, and the coalescence of their tendinous insertions is on the humerus.
- The supraspinatus and infraspinatus insert on the greater tuberosity and are innervated by the suprascapular nerve (C5, C6); the supraspinatus abducts and the infraspinatus externally rotates the humerus.
- The teres minor is supplied by the axillary nerve (C5) and inserts on the greater tuberosity; its main function is to externally rotate the humerus.
- The subscapularis is innervated by the upper and lower subscapular nerves (C5 through C7), inserts on the lesser tuberosity, and internally rotates the humerus.
- The axillary nerve exits the quadrangular space and wraps around the humerus to innervate the deltoid and is identifiable approximately 5 cm distal to the anterolateral corner of the acromion.
- Full-thickness RC tears may be associated with significant retraction of the tendon; alteration of the normal anatomy and atrophy of the tendons are related to the chronicity of the tear and injury to the suprascapular nerve.

PROCEDURES

Arthroscopic Rotator Cuff Repair

- May be performed in the lateral decubitus or beach chair position.
- Standard portals are established, including posterior, posterolateral, anterior, and anterolateral (Figure 12-3).
- Diagnostic arthroscopy is performed to assess for any intra-articular glenohumeral pathology, which is addressed as necessary. Specifically, the biceps tendon should be evaluated, because it may cause concomitant pain in RC pathology.
- Subacromial bursectomy and acromioplasty are performed (see Chapter 11) with release of coracoacromial ligament except in massive, irreparable tears. In larger tears, release of the coracoacromial ligament may result in superior migration and anterior superior escape of the humeral head.[21]
- The torn RC tendon is visualized, débrided, and mobilized.
- Specially designed suture anchors are utilized to repair the tendon either in a single- or double-row technique (Figure 12-4); anatomic restoration of the footprint must be achieved to provide an optimal healing environment and allow early range of motion. Newer double-row fixation techniques allow fixation equivalent to the transosseus suture fixation achieved in open repairs.
- For patients with massive RC tears, a partial repair may improve function, while isolated débridement, subacromial decompression, and biceps tenotomy may relieve pain.

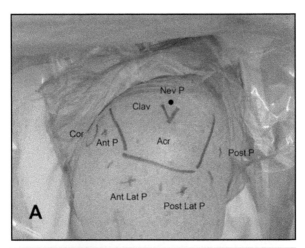

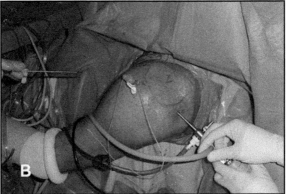

Figure 12-3. (A) Intraoperative photograph demonstrating the skin landmarks and arthroscopic portal placement for rotator cuff repair. Acr=acromion, Ant Lat P=anterolateral portal, Ant P=anterior portal, Clav=clavicle, Cor=coracoid, Nev P=Neviaser portal, Post Lat P=posterolateral portal, and Post P=posterior portal. (B) Intraoperative photograph of an arthroscopic rotator cuff repair utilizing the posterior portal for visualization and the anterolateral portal for placement of suture anchors.

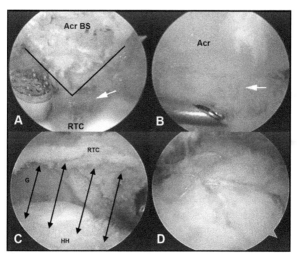

Figure 12-4. Intraoperative arthroscopic images. (A) A large acromial bone spur (Acr BS) with a narrowed subacromial space (white arrow) and fraying of the underlying rotator cuff tendon (RTC). (B) Arthroscopic acromioplasty with the utilization of an arthroscopic burr from the lateral portal to create a flat contour to the acromion with resultant increase in the subacromial space (white arrow). (C) A full-thickness RC tear with black arrows marking the retraction of the supraspinatus tendon (RTC) and exposed glenoid (G) and humeral head (HH). (D) Restoration of the RC footprint after arthroscopic repair using a double-row technique with suture anchors.

Open and Mini-Open Rotator Cuff Repair

Previous techniques for a formal open approach involved a larger incision with release of the deltoid from the acromion to provide direct visualization for preparation and repair of the RC. This technique evolved to a more minimally invasive or mini-open (arthroscopically assisted) approach. Mini-open procedures are completed utilizing an arthroscope for débridement of the tendon, placing initial sutures in the RC, and/or preparation of the foot-print. A small lateral deltoid splint is utilized and suture anchors or a transosseous repair is undertaken.

REHABILITATION

- Patients undergoing subacromial decompression with or without small RC repair participate in early range of motion and strengthening exercises with a physical therapist.
- The shoulder of patients with medium-sized RC repairs is immobilized for 2 weeks prior to initiation of physical therapy.
- The shoulder of patients with large RC repairs or poor tissue quality is immobilized and active range of motion is initiated at 6 weeks, followed by strengthening at 10 weeks.
- Complete recovery most commonly takes 4 to 6 months, although this varies.

OUTCOMES

Nonoperative Results

- The outcome and natural history of RC tears contin-ues to be debated. Studies have shown pain relief (62% to 74%) with nonoperative modalities, how-ever, restoration of strength was limited.[22,23] A natu-ral history of progression has been noted, with 52% of full-thickness tears increasing in size (as com-pared to 8% of partial-thickness tears).[24] Patients treated nonoperatively should be monitored clini-cally for progression of the tear. If progression is suspected, a new MRI study can be used to confirm clinical examination findings and document any changes.

- Both NSAIDs and injections are significantly superior to placebo for reducing pain and demonstrate similar efficacies in treating shoulder pain and RC tendinitis in randomized, controlled trials.[25,26]
- Physical therapy and exercise have shown consistently good results for improvement of pain and some increased function, but maintenance of strength has been less certain.
- Most clinicians recommend an initial trial of nonoperative management for patients with impingement, certain partial-thickness tears, and irreparable massive RC tears in the elderly.
- Although nonoperative treatment may be effective in reducing inflammation, decreasing pain, and restoring function in impingement and some partial-thickness tears, it may have limited use in restoring strength and function in full-thickness tears secondary to the complete discontinuity of the tendon.

Operative Results

- Overall success rates have been reported to be 75% to 86% for relief of impingement symptoms.[27,28] Two randomized trials demonstrated a significant difference favoring subacromial decompression over physical therapy, while one showed no difference.[29]
- Previously, most partial tears of greater than 50% thickness were treated with débridement alone; however, new research demonstrates improved outcomes with repair. Good to excellent results have been reported with operative repair of partial-thickness RC tears in 50% to 89% of patients.[30-32]
- Arthroscopic treatment of full-thickness tears has yielded excellent results with a 78% to 80% success rate, 95% to 98.6% patient satisfaction, and 95.5%

of patients stating that they would have the procedure performed again.[33,34]

- For massive RC tears, good results with greater than
  80% satisfaction have been attained following débridement and subacromial decompression alone;
  in younger individuals with a higher level of activity
  requirement, a tendon transfer may be performed,
  with early data showing satisfactory outcomes.[35,36]

POTENTIAL COMPLICATIONS[37,38]

- Failure of repair (6%)
- Stiffness (4%)
- Neurovascular damage (1%)
- Infection (greater than 1%)
- Complications requiring reoperation occur at similar
  rates following use of mini-open and arthroscopic
  techniques[38]
- Deltoid dehiscence may occur after open repair

REFERENCES

1. Praemer AFS, Rice D. *Musculoskeletal Conditions in the United States*. 2nd ed. Rosemont, IL: American Academy of Orthopaedic Surgeons; 1999.

2. Fukuda H. Partial-thickness rotator cuff tears: a modern view on Codman's classic. *J Shoulder Elbow Surg*. 2000; 9(2):163-168.

3. Milgrom C, Schaffler M, Gilbert S, van Holsbeeck M. Rotator-cuff changes in asymptomatic adults. The effect of age, hand dominance and gender. *J Bone Joint Surg Br*. 1995;77(2):296-298.

4. Sher JS, Uribe JW, Posada A, Murphy BJ, Zlatkin MB. Abnormal findings on magnetic resonance images of asymptomatic shoulders. *J Bone Joint Surg Am*. 1995;77(1): 10-15.

5. Yamamoto A, Takagishi K, Osawa T, et al. Prevalence and risk factors of a rotator cuff tear in the general population. *J Shoulder Elbow Surg*. 2010;19(1):116-120.

6. Kim HM, Teefey SA, Zelig A, Galatz LM, Keener JD, Yamaguchi K. Shoulder strength in asymptomatic individuals with intact compared with torn rotator cuffs. *J Bone Joint Surg Am.* 2009;91(2):289-296.

7. Ogata S, Uhthoff HK. Acromial enthesopathy and rotator cuff tear. A radiologic and histologic postmortem investigation of the coracoacromial arch. *Clin Orthop Relat Res.* 1990;254:39-48.

8. Neer CS 2nd. Impingement lesions. *Clin Orthop Relat Res.* 1983;173:70-77.

9. Gotoh M, Hamada K, Yamakawa H, Inoue A, Fukuda H. Increased substance P in subacromial bursa and shoulder pain in rotator cuff diseases. *J Orthop Res.* 1998;16(5):618-621.

10. Gotoh M, Hamada K, Yamakawa H, et al. Interleukin-1-induced glenohumeral synovitis and shoulder pain in rotator cuff diseases. *J Orthop Res.* 2002;20(6): 1365-1371.

11. Walch G, Liotard JP, Boileau P, Noel E. [Postero-superior glenoid impingement. Another impingement of the shoulder]. *J Radiol.* 1993;74(1):47-50.

12. Goutallier D, Postel JM, Bernageau J, Lavau L, Voisin MC. Fatty muscle degeneration in cuff ruptures. Pre- and post-operative evaluation by CT scan. *Clin Orthop Relat Res.* 1994;304:78-83.

13. De Jesus JO, Parker L, Frangos AJ, Nazarian LN. Accuracy of MRI, MR arthrography, and ultrasound in the diagnosis of rotator cuff tears: a meta-analysis. *AJR Am J Roentgenol.* 2009;192(6):1701-1707.

14. Fotiadou AN, Vlychou M, Papadopoulos P, Karataglis DS, Palladas P, Fezoulidis IV. Ultrasonography of symptomatic rotator cuff tears compared with MR imaging and surgery. *Eur J Radiol.* 2008;68(1):174-179.

15. Teefey SA, Rubin DA, Middleton WD, Hildebolt CF, Leibold RA, Yamaguchi K. Detection and quantification of rotator cuff tears. Comparison of ultrasonographic, magnetic resonance imaging, and arthroscopic findings in seventy-one consecutive cases. *J Bone Joint Surg Am.* 2004;86-A(4):708-716.

16. Waldt S, Bruegel M, Mueller D, et al. Rotator cuff tears: assessment with MR arthrography in 275 patients with arthroscopic correlation. *Eur Radiol.* 2007;17(2): 491-498.

17. Chen MJ, Lew HL, Hsu TC, et al. Ultrasound-guided shoulder injections in the treatment of subacromial bursitis. *Am J Phys Med Rehabil*. 2006;85(1):31-35.

18. Eustace JA, Brophy DP, Gibney RP, Bresnihan B, FitzGerald O. Comparison of the accuracy of steroid placement with clinical outcome in patients with shoulder symptoms. *Ann Rheum Dis*. 1997;56(1):59-63.

19. Henkus HE, Cobben LP, Coerkamp EG, Nelissen RG, van Arkel ER. The accuracy of subacromial injections: a prospective randomized magnetic resonance imaging study. *Arthroscopy*. 2006;22(3):277-282.

20. Marx RG, Koulouvaris P, Chu SK, Levy BA. Indications for surgery in clinical outcome studies of rotator cuff repair. *Clin Orthop Relat Res*. 2009;467(2):450-456.

21. Lafosse L. Arthroscopic Repair of rotator cuff tears. In: Warner JJP, Iannotti JP, Flatow EL, eds. *Complex and Revision Problems in Shoulder Surgery*. 2nd ed. Philadelphia, PA: Lippincott Williams and Wilkins; 2005:161-187.

22. Bokor DJ, Hawkins RJ, Huckell GH, Angelo RL, Schickendantz MS. Results of nonoperative management of full-thickness tears of the rotator cuff. *Clin Orthop Relat Res*. 1993;294:103-110.

23. Wirth MA, Basamania C, Rockwood CA Jr. Nonoperative management of full-thickness tears of the rotator cuff. *Orthop Clin North Am*. 1997;28(1):59-67.

24. Yamaguchi K, Ditsios K, Middleton WD, Hildebolt CF, Galatz LM, Teefey SA. The demographic and morphological features of rotator cuff disease. A comparison of asymptomatic and symptomatic shoulders. *J Bone Joint Surg Am*. 2006;88(8):1699-1704.

25. Green SBR, Hetrick S. Physiotherapy interventions for shoulder pain. *Cochrane Database Syst Rev*. 2003;(2):CD004258.

26. Petri M, Dobrow R, Neiman R, Whiting-O'Keefe Q, Seaman WE. Randomized, double-blind, placebo-controlled study of the treatment of the painful shoulder. *Arthritis Rheum*. 1987;30(9):1040-1045.

27. Hawkins RJ, Plancher KD, Saddemi SR, Brezenoff LS, Moor JT. Arthroscopic subacromial decompression. *J Shoulder Elbow Surg*. 2001;10(3):225-230.

28. Patel VR, Singh D, Calvert PT, Bayley JI. Arthroscopic subacromial decompression: results and factors affecting outcome. *J Shoulder Elbow Surg.* 1999;8(3):231-237.

29. Brox JI, Gjengedal E, Uppheim G, et al. Arthroscopic surgery versus supervised exercises in patients with rotator cuff disease (stage II impingement syndrome): a prospective, randomized, controlled study in 125 patients with a 2½-year follow-up. *J Shoulder Elbow Surg.* 1999;8(2):102-111.

30. Budoff JE, Nirschl RP, Guidi EJ. Debridement of partial-thickness tears of the rotator cuff without acromioplasty. Long-term follow-up and review of the literature. *J Bone Joint Surg Am.* 1998;80(5):733-748.

31. Ogilvie-Harris DJ, Wiley AM. Arthroscopic surgery of the shoulder. A general appraisal. *J Bone Joint Surg Br.* 1986;68(2):201-207.

32. Snyder SJ, Pachelli AF, Del Pizzo W, Friedman MJ, Ferkel RD, Pattee G. Partial thickness rotator cuff tears: results of arthroscopic treatment. *Arthroscopy.* 1991;7(1):1-7.

33. Bennett WF. Arthroscopic repair of massive rotator cuff tears: a prospective cohort with 2- to 4-year follow-up. *Arthroscopy.* 2003;19(4):380-390.

34. Cofield RH, Parvizi J, Hoffmeyer PJ, Lanzer WL, Ilstrup DM, Rowland CM. Surgical repair of chronic rotator cuff tears. A prospective long-term study. *J Bone Joint Surg Am.* 2001;83-A(1):71-77.

35. Iannotti JP, Hennigan S, Herzog R, et al. Latissimus dorsi tendon transfer for irreparable posterosuperior rotator cuff tears. Factors affecting outcome. *J Bone Joint Surg Am.* 2006;88(2):342-348.

36. Gartsman GM. Massive, irreparable tears of the rotator cuff. Results of operative debridement and subacromial decompression. *J Bone Joint Surg Am.* 1997;79(5):715-721.

37. Mansat P, Cofield RH, Kersten TE, Rowland CM. Complications of rotator cuff repair. *Orthop Clin North Am.* 1997;28(2):205-213.

38. Morse K, Davis AD, Afra R, Kaye EK, Schepsis A, Voloshin I. Arthroscopic versus mini-open rotator cuff repair: a comprehensive review and meta-analysis. *Am J Sports Med.* 2008;36(9):1824-1828.

Relevant Review Articles

Green A. Chronic massive rotator cuff tears: evaluation and management. *J Am Acad Orthop Surg.* 2003;11(5): 321-331.

Wolff AB, Sethi P, Sutton KM, Covey AS, Magit DP, Medvecky M. Partial-thickness rotator cuff tears. *J Am Acad Orthop Surg.* 2006;14(13):715-725.

CHAPTER 13 | ADHESIVE CAPSULITIS

Brent A. Ponce, MD;
Trent J. Wilson, MD;
Hinrich J. D. Heuer; and
Peter J. Millett, MD, MSc

MECHANISM OF INJURY/ PATHOPHYSIOLOGY

Adhesive capsulitis, or frozen shoulder, is a common shoulder disorder that is characterized by pain and loss of both active and passive motion. It is generally a self-limiting condition with a natural history lasting 1 to 3 years. While the etiology is unknown, adhesive capsulitis is associated with the following factors:

- Female gender
- Middle age (generally between 40 to 60 years)
- Medical conditions
    - Diabetes (affects people with diabetes at a rate 2 to 4 times higher than for the general population)
    - Thyroid disorders
    - Cardiac disease
    - Pulmonary disease
    - Surgery (eg, shoulder, cardiac, neurosurgery)
    - Dupuytren's disease
    - Parkinson's disease

227

Rohde RS, Millett PJ, eds.
*Evaluation and Management
of Common Upper Extremity Disorders:
A Practical Handbook* (pp 227-240).
© 2011 Taylor & Francis Group.

- □ Hyperlipidemia
- □ Low bone mineral density
- Trauma
    - □ Low- or high-energy injury of the shoulder (initiates inflammatory cascade)
    - □ Period of long immobilization (contributes to shoulder stiffness)
    - □ Concomitant ipsilateral upper extremity injuries such as distal radius fractures or elbow injuries
- Associated shoulder disease
    - □ Rotator cuff tear
    - □ Biceps tendinitis
    - □ Calcific tendinitis

KEY HISTORY POINTS

Symptoms include pain and loss of both active and passive motion of the shoulder. Loss of internal rotation is frequently present early in the course. In women, this may be manifested initially with difficulty fastening a brassiere. Men may complain that it is difficult to tuck in the back of a shirt or reach into a back pants pocket.

- Pain typically is worse at night and with extremes of motion. People usually describe the pain as having a gradual onset that is sometimes precipitated by a seemingly minor event.
- Pain usually is over the deltoid and may radiate toward the forearm.
- Gradually increasing pain and dysfunction can mimic rotator cuff pathology and must be evaluated carefully.
- This condition may affect up to 20% of people with diabetes and 5% of the general population.
- Bilateral involvement can occur in up to 50% of cases.

- Physicians should take a careful history of related risk factors.

There are 3 clinical stages: Inflammatory (or freezing), frozen, and thawing (or resolving). The total course typically lasts around 30 months, but symptoms might not resolve for up to 42 months.

- The **inflammatory** stage may last from 10 to 36 weeks. Pain frequently is poorly controlled with nonsteroidal anti-inflammatory drugs (NSAIDs).
- The **frozen** stage occurs 4 to 12 months after the onset of symptoms. Although pain is improved at rest, it is exacerbated with extreme motion. Examination demonstrates notable loss of motion.
- The **thawing** stage is associated with spontaneous increased range of motion. Some patients may have persistent symptoms refractory to time and conservative management.

KEY EXAMINATION POINTS

As with other upper extremity conditions, evaluation from the neck to the fingertips is recommended. Thorough examination of the shoulder and surrounding structures must be done to eliminate other pathology. Evaluate and document active and passive ranges of motion at every visit to assess progress. The following examination findings are commonly observed in adhesive capsulitis cases:

- Decrease in both active and passive motion with firm motion endpoints due to fibrotic tight capsule (as opposed to soft endpoints from muscular guarding or pain)
- Decreased internal and external rotation of maximally abducted shoulder (compared to contralateral shoulder)
- Absence of asymmetric atrophy (neurologic process), masses (possible tumor), swelling, erythema

(infection), scapular winging (may be compensa-
tory or long thoracic nerve palsy), crepitation
(fracture)

ADDITIONAL TESTING OR IMAGING

Diagnosis is based upon history and clinical examination rather than diagnostic tests. However, some tests
may be used as adjuncts in confirming the diagnosis
and evaluating the effectiveness of treatment. These tests
include the following:

- **Radiographs** of the shoulder should be obtained
  on all patients suspected of adhesive capsulitis.
  This includes anteroposterior films in external
  and internal rotation, a supraspinatus outlet view,
  and an axillary view. Films will help exclude
  tumors, osteoarthritis, calcific tendinitis, and
  fractures.
- **Lidocaine injection test:** 10 mL of lidocaine injected into the subacromial space will decrease
  pain from a possible rotator cuff lesion; this
  injection will not provide significant relief in the
  frozen shoulder and therefore can help differentiate
  between these 2 causes of motion loss.
- **Arthrography** demonstrates decreased joint volume
  compared to other shoulder conditions and screens
  for rotator cuff tears. Cuomo and colleagues consider arthrography a standard diagnostic technique
  to confirm frozen shoulder, but it is not absolutely
  mandatory for diagnosis.[1]
- **Magnetic resonance imaging** frequently is inter-
  preted as normal. Coracohumeral ligament and
  rotator interval thickening may be identified.
- **Laboratory tests** typically are normal except in
  cases associated with diabetes, thyroid disease, or
  hyperlipidemia; ordering laboratory tests should be
  considered on a case-by-case basis.

Treatment Options: Nonoperative

Early efforts should be made to identify patients at increased risk of developing adhesive capsulitis and intervention initiated. In addition, it is crucial to avoid the misdiagnosis of other shoulder disorders. Surgery to address other conditions (eg, impingement, rotator cuff tear) may worsen the pain and dysfunction associated with adhesive capsulitis. Although observation is the mainstay treatment for adhesive capsulitis, there are some nonoperative measures that may help with pain and dysfunction. It is also important to provide frequent reassurance to encourage patients through the often prolonged course of the disease.

- Oral agents
    - Little evidence to confirm efficacy of NSAIDs
    - Little evidence to support routine use of oral corticosteroids[2]
    - Narcotics should be avoided
- Injection
    - Intra-articular corticosteroid injections provide pain relief which may facilitate rehabilitation[3]
- Physical therapy
    - An active assisted range of motion program with gentle, passive stretching exercises is helpful. These exercises should be performed 4 to 5 times per day. Heat before and ice after therapy may facilitate flexibility and reduce inflammation.
- Capsular distension or brisement (injection of fluid to disrupt joint capsule) has demonstrated variable results; it may be considered early in the course of disease prior to significant capsular thickening.[4]

TREATMENT OPTIONS: OPERATIVE

Surgical intervention, either open or arthroscopic, aims to release the contracted tissue to gain movement and relieve pain.

- Indications for manipulation under anesthesia (MUA) are controversial, but MUA has been shown to decrease time to return to normal range of motion. MUA should be considered only after 3 to 6 months of unsuccessful supervised physical therapy.
- Neither MUA nor any surgical interventions should be considered while the patient is experiencing the severe pain seen during the inflammatory stage because of the potential to worsen symptoms. Regional anesthesia, blocks, and indwelling catheters have been used with excellent results. MUA may be performed independently or in conjunction with arthroscopic release.
- Arthroscopic capsular release is the mainstay of surgical intervention and can be performed before or after MUA. If a subacromial bursectomy is performed, the acromioplasty should be limited to reduce bleeding and scar formation.
- Open release is recommended only after failed arthroscopic capsular release or when adhesions are primarily extra-articular.

SURGICAL ANATOMY

- Rotator interval: Triangular space between supraspinatus and subscapularis rotator cuff tendons and base of coracoid (Figure 13-1)
- Middle glenohumeral ligament: Deep to intra-articular portion of subscapularis; most variable of glenohumeral ligaments (Figure 13-2)

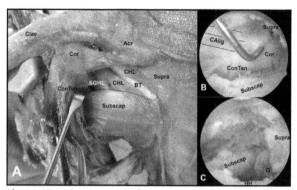

Figure 13-1. Rotator interval. (A) Picture of a dissected left shoulder viewing the rotator interval (shadowed area) with the superior glenohumeral ligament (SGHL), coracohumeral ligament (CHL), and biceps tendon (BT). (B) Arthroscopic picture viewing out of the joint through the rotator interval onto the coracoid (Cor). (C) Arthroscopic view from the subacromial space through the rotator interval onto the glenoid. Acr=acromion, CAlig=coracoacromial ligament, Clav=clavicle, ConTen=conjoined tendon, G=glenoid, HH=humeral head, Subscap=subscapularis, Supra=supraspinatus.

- Inferior glenohumeral ligament: Anterior and posterior bands attach to glenoid and humerus in a hammock-like fashion; this provides restraint to anterior translation when the arm is in an abducted and externally rotated position
- Joint capsule: Deepest layer of the rotator cuff

PROCEDURES

- Arthroscopic capsular release (Figure 13-3)
    - General anesthesia is induced following placement of an interscalene block with or without an indwelling catheter for better postoperative pain control and to facilitate therapy postoperatively.

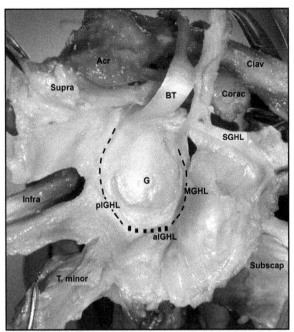

Figure 13-2. Picture of dissected left shoulder viewing from lateral onto the glenoid with humerus removed. The thin dotted lines at the anterior and posterior capsulolabral junction indicate where an arthroscopic release should be made. If the shoulder is still tight after releasing along these lines, further release can be made along the thick dotted line at the inferior capsulolabral junction, but special care should be taken to avoid damaging the axillary nerve. Acr=acromion, a/pIGHL=anterior and posterior inferior glenohumeral ligament, BT=biceps tendon, Clav=clavicle, Corac=coracoid, G=glenoid, Infra=infraspinatus muscle, MGHL=middle glenohumeral ligament, SGHL=superior glenohumeral ligament, Subscap=subscapularis muscle, Supra=supraspinatus muscle, T. minor=teres minor muscle.

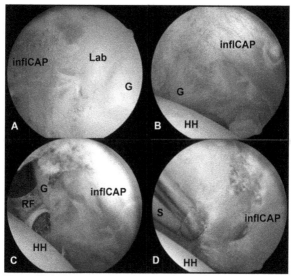

Figure 13-3. Intraoperative pictures of an arthroscopic capsular release of a left shoulder. (A) Anterior inflamed capsule (inflCAP). (B) Posterior inflamed capsule. (C) Resection of inflamed capsule with radio frequency ablation device (RF). (D) Further resection of capsule with shaver (S). G=glenoid, HH=humeral head, Lab=labrum.

- □ The patient is positioned in a beach chair or lateral decubitus position.
- □ The shoulder is examined under anesthesia and preoperative range of motion measurements are determined.
- □ Manipulation can be performed before, during, or after arthroscopy.
- □ Reduced volume may increase difficulty to enter the joint with the arthroscope; injection with normal saline solution can be performed to distend the joint.

- Standard posterior and anterior arthroscopy portals are established and thorough arthroscopic examination is performed. (For details, see Chapters 12 and 14.)
- The biceps tendon and upper edge of the subscapularis are identified. Capsular release begins at the rotator interval using an arthroscopic radio frequency ablating device until the fibers of the conjoined tendon are seen running longitudinally. This division releases the coracohumeral ligament and anterosuperior capsule, which often inhibit external rotation.
- Continual use of the radio frequency device is limited to avoid thermal necrosis of tissues (eg, cartilage, capsule, axillary nerve). The intra-articular cannula is kept open to improve fluid egress from the joint and reduce joint temperatures.
- The anterior capsule/middle glenohumeral ligament over the subscapularis tendon is released down to and below the anterior band of the glenohumeral ligament to reopen the subscapularis recess. Performing the release close to the glenoid rim inferiorly decreases the risk of axillary nerve injury; the nerve may be only 12.4 mm from the glenoid rim at the 6 o'clock position.[5]
- Access to release the inferior capsule may be facilitated by using a postero-inferior portal.
- The camera is moved from the posterior viewing portal to the anterosuperior portal, and the radio frequency device is inserted through the posterior portal. Posterior release through the posterior band of the inferior glenohumeral ligament is performed.
- Some patients with adhesive capsulitis secondary to a previous operation or fracture may have extensive subacromial scarring that mandates débridement.

- □ Manipulation after release begins with the surgeon's hands as near the shoulder as possible (to avoid a long lever arm and increased risk of creating a fracture in osteopenic patients). The shoulder is flexed gently, then abducted, externally rotated, and internally rotated. Following gradual capsular release, final range of motion measurements are assessed.
- Open release
  - □ Advantages include direct visualization of contracted structures, but disadvantages include increased postoperative pain.
  - □ Structures released include subacromial and subdeltoid adhesions, coracohumeral ligament, rotator interval, perilabral tissues, and subscapularis.
  - □ General anesthesia and interscalene block with or without catheter are used.
  - □ A deltopectoral approach is used.
  - □ Adhesions between the deltoid and the humerus are released; care is taken to protect the axillary nerve.
  - □ The coracoacromial ligament is incised, and scarring within the subacromial space is débrided. The underlying rotator cuff is identified and protected.
  - □ Dissection continues deep to the conjoined tendon, and after dissection of the supraspinatus and subscapularis from the coracoid, the coracohumeral ligament and the rotator interval are released.
  - □ Persistent tightness in external rotation at this point mandates subscapularis tenotomy or Z-lengthening and excision of the anterior capsule. This is repaired loosely at the end of the case using nonabsorbable sutures. Each centimeter of length gained increases external rotation by approximately 20 degrees.

□ If abduction and internal rotation still are limited, the inferior and posterior capsule should
be released.

REHABILITATION

Immediate gentle and full range of motion without
limitations or restrictions are essential. It is often helpful
for the surgeon or therapist to demonstrate to the patient
the marked improvement in range of motion in the recovery room so the patient can better understand postoperative expectations.

- Ideally, rehabilitation should be supervised and
directed by the therapist initially (consider 5 therapy
sessions a week for the first 2 weeks) to push the
patient through postoperative pain in order to maintain the gains obtained intraoperatively.
- A sling is necessary only while the extremity remains anesthetized because the patient will have
limited control. It is removed on postoperative
day 1 to allow for activities of daily living.

OUTCOMES

- Nonoperative treatment (stretching program)
    □ In one series, a 90% satisfaction rate was
    obtained with nonoperative treatment; only
    7% of patients required a manipulation or
    capsular release. Despite favorable results,
    many patients continued to report pain and
    decreased motion compared to the unaffected
    shoulder.[6]
- Manipulation versus intra-articular distension with
Marcaine (bupivacaine hydrochloride) and steroid
or radio-opaque saline solution (ie, brisement
procedure)

□ No difference has been noted with regard to pain reduction and function between patients who underwent MUA, in-office joint distension, or hydraulic distension using fluoroscopic guidance.[7-9]
- Manipulation versus surgery
  □ In a comparison of patients who underwent MUA or arthroscopic release, patients achieved a similar range of movement but less pain and overall better function following surgical release 2 to 5 years after surgery.[10]

POTENTIAL COMPLICATIONS

Complications associated with treatment of adhesive capsulitis usually are iatrogenic and are the result of the treatment used. Potential complications include:
- Humerus or glenoid fracture
- Glenohumeral dislocation
- Rotator cuff tears
- Labral detachment
- Brachial plexus stretch injury
- Axillary nerve injuries
- Recurrent stiffness

REFERENCES

1. Cuomo F, Flatow EL, Schneider JA, Bishop JY. Idiopathic and diabetic stiff shoulder: decision-making and treatment. In: Warner JJP, Iannotti JP, Flatow EL, eds. *Complex and Revision Problems in Shoulder Surgery*. 2nd ed. Philadelphia, PA: Lippincott Williams and Wilkins; 2005:205-229.
2. Buchbinder R, Green S, Youd JM, Johnston RV. Oral steroids for adhesive capsulitis. *Cochrane Database Syst Rev.* 2006;18(4):CD006189.

3. Bal A, Eksioglu E, Gulec B, Aydog E, Gurcay E, Cakci A. Effectiveness of corticosteroid injection in adhesive capsulitis. *Clin Rehabil*. 2008;22(6):503-512.

4. Vad VB, Sakalkale D, Warren RE. The role of capsular distension in adhesive capsulits. *Arch Phys Med Rehabil*. 2003;84:1290-1292.

5. Price MR, Tillett ED, Acland RD, Nettleton GS. Determining the relationship of the axillary nerve of the shoulder joint capsule from an arthroscopic perspective. *J Bone Joint Surg Am*. 2004;8:2135-2142.

6. Griggs S, Ahn A, Green A. Idiopathic adhesive capsulitis: a prospective functional outcome study of non-operative treatment. *J Bone Joint Surg Am*. 2000;82:1398-1407.

7. Jacobs LG, Smith MG, Khan SA, Smith K, Joshi M. Manipulation or intra-articular steroids in the management of adhesive capsulitis of the shoulder? A prospective randomized trial. *J Shoulder Elbow Surg*. 2009;18(3): 348-353.

8. Quraishi NA, Johnston P, Bayer J, Crowe M, Chakrbarti AJ. Thawing the frozen shoulder: a randomized trail comparing manipulation under anesthesis with hydrodilatation. *J Bone Joint Surg Br*. 2007;89:1197-1200.

9. Sharma RK, Bajekal RA, Bhan S. Frozen shoulder syndrome. A comparison of hydraulic distension and manipulation. *Int Orthop*. 1993;17:275-278.

10. Ogilvie-Harris DJ, Biggs DJ, Fitsialos DP, MacKay M. The resistant frozen shoulder. Manipulation versus arthroscopic release. *Clin Orthop Relat Res*. 1995;319: 238-248.

Relevant Review Articles

Chambler AFW, Carr AJ. Aspects of current management: the role of surgery in frozen shoulder. *J Bone Joint Surg Br*. 2003;85(6):789-795.

Warner J, Answorth A, Marks P, Wong P. Frozen shoulder: diagnosis and management. *J Am Acad Orthop Surg*. 1997;5:130-140.

CHAPTER 14

SHOULDER INSTABILITY

James R. Romanowski, MD;
Danny P. Goel, MD, FRCSC; and
Jon J. P. Warner, MD

MECHANISM OF INJURY/ PATHOPHYSIOLOGY

Shoulder instability remains one of the most common orthopedic problems facing clinicians today. The term encompasses multiple diagnoses, and a thorough evaluation is necessary to define the underlying pathology and subsequently formulate a treatment plan. The spectrum of shoulder instability ranges from subtle subluxation of the humeral head within the glenoid to gross dislocation. The age of the patient at the time of initial dislocation, duration of symptoms (acute versus chronic), mechanism of injury (traumatic versus atraumatic), and direction of instability (unidirectional versus multidirectional) remain critical components that must be identified.

Mechanism of Injury

Traumatic

- **Anterior** shoulder dislocations typically result from injuries related to forceful abduction and external rotation of the upper extremity.

Rohde RS, Millett PJ, eds.
Evaluation and Management
of Common Upper Extremity Disorders:
A Practical Handbook (pp 241-270).
© 2011 Taylor & Francis Group.

- **Posterior** dislocations occur with a posteriorly directed force with the shoulder positioned in adduction, internal rotation, and forward flexion.
    □ Seizures and electrical shock also might precipitate a dislocation as the internal rotation moment of the subscapularis overpowers the posterior restraint of the infraspinatus and teres minor.

Atraumatic

- Multidirectional instability
    □ Connective tissue defects
        • Ehlers-Danlos syndrome
        • Marfan syndrome
    □ Repetitive microtrauma
    □ Swimming, pitching, volleyball, and other overhead-motion athletic activities
- Glenoid dysplasia

Pathophysiology

An understanding of shoulder anatomy is necessary for one to determine the underlying defects contributing to shoulder instability.

- The shoulder comprises 4 articulations: Glenohumeral, acromioclavicular, sternoclavicular, and scapulothoracic.
- Shoulder instability generally involves the glenohumeral joint.
- The joint is considered to have both static and dynamic components.
    □ **Static stabilizers**
        • The main contributors to static shoulder stability involve the ball-and-socket bony articulation, the labrum, which provides a soft-tissue cuff that deepens the socket, and the joint capsule.

- The capsular contribution to static stability may be defined further by focal condensations of collagen that provide additional restraint based on the position of the arm—superior glenohumeral ligament (SGHL), middle glenohumeral ligament (MGHL), and anterior and posterior bands of the inferior glenohumeral ligament (IGHL).
  - The SGHL provides resistance to inferior translation with the arm in neutral position.
  - The MGHL provides anterior restraint with increasing abduction angles, particularly at 45 degrees.
  - The anterior band of the IGHL is the primary capsular stabilizer for shoulder abduction at 90 degrees.
- **Dynamic stabilizers** include the long head of the biceps tendon, negative intra-articular pressure, and the surrounding musculature of the shoulder girdle—primarily the rotator cuff muscles (subscapularis, supraspinatus, infraspinatus, and teres minor). Additional muscles and ligamentous structures provide further support to the stability of the shoulder.

KEY HISTORY POINTS

- The position of the arm and direction of force during the initial injury can help determine the underlying structural damage in the setting of traumatic instability.
- The age of the patient at the time of initial dislocation should be noted. While younger patients have a higher recurrent dislocation rate, elderly patients have a higher incidence of associated rotator cuff tears.

- The number of dislocations can be used to guide treatment.
  - ☐ A single dislocation without recurrent instability may be treated nonoperatively, but multiple dislocations may be an indication for surgical intervention.
  - ☐ Inciting events for recurrent dislocation can predict degree of instability; dislocations that occur during sleep, while reaching for objects, or via other relatively low-energy mechanisms suggest increased instability.
  - ☐ Prior treatment modalities should be ascertained:
    - Immobilization
    - Physical therapy
    - Surgical intervention
      - ○ For patients who have had prior surgery, it is necessary to establish which procedures were performed as well as the implants used for the prior repair.

KEY EXAMINATION POINTS

A thorough examination requires visualization and evaluation of both upper extremities, including the neck. Bony and muscular contours as well as tenderness to palpation must be appreciated. Range of motion and the neurovascular status are evaluated. The strength of the rotator cuff and surrounding musculature of the shoulder girdle and arm should be documented to help rule out additional pathology (Table 14-1).

- Instability should not be confused with laxity. Laxity is an objective physical exam finding that may not be pathologic. This is in contrast to instability, which is a subjective finding described by the patient.

Table 14-1.
Shoulder Examination for Instability

Examination	Technique	Illustration	Grading	Significance
Range of motion	Examine in standing and supine positions. Forward flexion, scaption, abduction, and internal and external rotation are documented.		Compared bilaterally.	Deficiencies may suggest associated pathology such as rotator cuff tears or contractures.
Palpation	Patient is standing with the arm supported by the examiner.		Tenderness over the greater tuberosity, bicipital groove, joint line, and AC joint are noted.	Helps establish or rule out additional shoulder pathology.
Apprehension test	With the shoulder in 90 degrees of abduction, the arm is externally rotated.		Sensation of the humeral head dislocating anteriorly is considered positive.	Tests the compliance of the anterior joint capsule and anterior band of the inferior glenohumeral ligament.

(CONTINUED)

Table 14-1.
Shoulder Examination for Instability (continued)

Examination	Technique	Illustration	Grading	Significance
Jobe relocation test	When the apprehension test is positive, a posterior force is directed on the proximal humerus.		Decreased apprehension with the posterior force is considered a positive test.	Clinically recreates the function of the anterior joint capsule and the inferior glenohumeral ligament.
Posterior translation	Posterior translation is tested with the arm in slight abduction and neutral rotation. The humeral head is palpated and a posterior force is applied.		Grade 0: No translation to glenoid rim. Grade 1+: Translation to glenoid rim. Grade 2+: Humeral head dislocated, but spontaneously reduces. Grade 3+: Humeral head remains dislocated.	Essential to compare to the asymptomatic side as normal patients may exhibit subluxation.

(CONTINUED)

Table 14-1.
Shoulder Examination for Instability (continued)

Examination	Technique	Illustration	Grading	Significance
Sulcus sign	With the patient seated, the upper extremity is positioned in 0 degrees abduction and 0 degrees external rotation. An inferior force is directed on the distal humerus. The test is repeated with the arm externally rotated to 90 degrees.		Grade 0: No translation to glenoid rim. Grade 1+: Translation to glenoid rim. Grade 2+: Humeral head dislocated, but spontaneously reduces. Grade 3+: Humeral head remains dislocated.	Increased translation at neutral, but normalizes with external rotation suggests a rotator interval (superior glenohumeral ligament) lesion. Increased translation at both 0 and 90 degrees represents multi-directional instability.

- Anterior
    - Apprehension test
    - Jobe relocation test
- Posterior
    - Jerk test
    - Kim test
- Inferior
    - A sulcus sign isolated to the arm in neutral rotation indicates a deficiency in the rotator interval, including the SGHL.
    - Failure of the sulcus sign to correct with external rotation implies multidirectional instability.
- Bidirectional instability is that noted in 2 directions
- Multidirectional instability is global
- Assess collagen laxity at other joints (Beighton signs)[1]
    - Thumb abduction (Figure 14-1)
    - Metacarpophalangeal middle hyperextension
    - Elbow hyperextension
    - Knee hyperextension
    - Palm to floor
- The status of the rotator cuff must be determined. Although rarely injured in adolescent shoulder dislocations, it commonly is injured in older patients with traumatic instability.

ADDITIONAL TESTING OR IMAGING

Imaging contributes critical information during the evaluation of patients with shoulder instability. Both bony and soft-tissue constraints may be affected; conservative and surgical managements are based on the competency of these tissues.

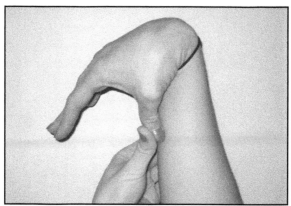

Figure 14-1. Collagen laxity demonstrated by hyperabduction of the thumb.

Each modality provides important information regarding the underlying pathology contributing to shoulder instability. All patients should be studied with plain radiographs at a minimum. Chronic, recurrent dislocators are best served with the addition of computed tomography (CT) arthrogram, as bony involvement is often a key contributor to the instability. Magnetic resonance imaging (MRI) is a reasonable study for the first-time dislocator when plain films suggest preservation of the bony surfaces.

Plain Radiographs

True anteroposterior (in the plane of the scapula) and axillary radiographs are required during the initial evaluation of patients with shoulder instability. Given the traumatic nature of most shoulder dislocations, the presence of fractures and static dislocations must be excluded. Additional views may help further define the underlying pathology and include the West Point axillary (anterior-inferior glenoid Bankart fractures), Garth (glenoid rim fractures), and Stryker Notch (Hill-Sachs lesions) views.

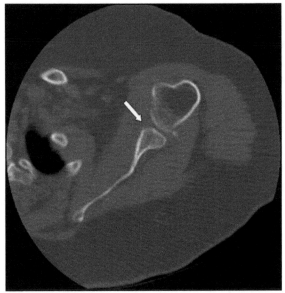

Figure 14-2. Axial CT scan of the glenohumeral joint. Anterior Bankart lesion (white arrow) is demonstrated with loss of glenoid bone.

Computed Tomography Scan

When plain radiographs suggest bony damage, a CT scan is helpful to define the lesion (Figure 14-2). This modality is particularly important for patients with recurrent dislocations. Coronal, sagittal, and axial sequences are required. The addition of intra-articular contrast helps further define the glenohumeral contours. Furthermore, 3-dimensional reconstructions provide valuable insight into the overall bony deformity (Figure 14-3).

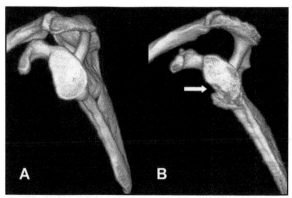

Figure 14-3. CT scan of the scapula with 3-D reconstructions. Normal glenoid (A) is compared to a glenoid (B) with a large anterior Bankart lesion (white arrow).

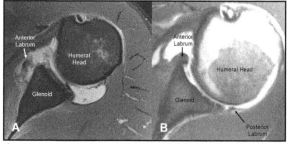

Figure 14-4. T2 axial MRI. (A) Anterior labral tear. (B) Posterior labral tear.

Magnetic Resonance Imaging

MRI allows for detailed assessment of the soft-tissue constraints of the shoulder (Figure 14-4). Intra-articular contrast is not necessary for acute injuries, as the joint is filled with a hematoma.

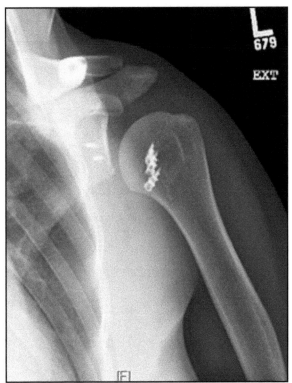

Figure 14-5. Plain anteroposterior radiograph of the shoulder. Note the inferior subluxation of the humeral head within the glenoid.

Electromyography

Electromyography is rarely necessary unless clinical and radiographic findings suggest nerve damage. Static inferior subluxation of the humeral head on the glenoid as well as atrophy and neurologic complaints involving the upper extremity imply nerve damage (Figure 14-5).

TREATMENT OPTIONS: NONOPERATIVE

Nonoperative intervention is a reasonable approach for the initial treatment of most first-time dislocators as well as chronic symptoms of subluxation or multidirectional instability. Defining the underlying pathology is critical in guiding the course of treatment.

Sling Immobilization

This should be the initial treatment after reduction of an acute shoulder dislocation.

- Immediate immobilization (within 24 hours of injury) in 10 degrees of external rotation for initial anterior dislocations has been shown to decrease the recurrence rate from 42% to 26%.[2]
- The duration of sling use has no significant effect on recurrence rates.[3]
- The sling is weaned as the pain resolves.
- Young contact athletes are at particular risk of recurrence, and the outcomes of conservative modalities should be discussed with the patient.
    - For patients younger than 40 years, 43% remained stable after initial dislocation with nonoperative management.[4] Seven percent redislocated once, and 50% had multiple redislocations.

Activity Modification

- Positions and activities that create situations of instability are avoided.

Functional Bracing

- Patients recovering from an initial dislocation, particularly overhead-throwing athletes, may benefit from bracing that limits abduction and external rotation. This may allow the athlete to complete participation in the athletic season and delay surgical intervention.

Physical Therapy

- Physical therapy is beneficial when the dislocation is associated with traumatic anterior instability. Initial focus (0 to 4 weeks) is avoidance of shoulder positioning that recreates the instability while maintaining range of motion.
- Isotonic rotator cuff and periscapular strengthening is initiated after 4 weeks, with progression to isokinetic exercises. Players usually are allowed to return to play once full range of motion is achieved and the strength is re-established.
- In cases of chronic subluxation or multidirectional instability, a regimen focused on scapular stabilization, proprioceptive training, and rotator cuff strengthening usually prevents the need for surgical intervention.[5]

TREATMENT OPTIONS: OPERATIVE

Indications for surgical management of shoulder instability include failure of conservative measures, recurrent dislocations, instability or symptomatic subluxation that interferes with activities of daily living, large bony Bankart lesions, and young age—particularly for first-time anterior shoulder dislocations. Damage isolated to soft tissue often may be addressed arthroscopically. More extensive damage with involvement of the glenoid may require bony reconstruction.

- Surgical intervention is based upon accurate identification of the underlying pathology. Young (ie, less than 24 years of age) first-time anterior dislocators have demonstrated the following:

- ▫ Antero-inferior Bankart lesion in 97%[6]
- ▫ Hill-Sachs lesion in 47% to 89%[7]
- ▫ Recurrent instability in 90% of patients treated nonoperatively
- Arthroscopy
  - ▫ Immediate arthroscopic stabilization in patients less than 30 years of age has a 16% redislocation rate when compared to a 47% rate with rehabilitation alone.[8]
  - ▫ Open procedures have been considered the gold standard for years; however, the evolution of arthroscopy has enabled surgeons to achieve equivalent results in the setting of isolated soft-tissue pathology.[9]
- **Open procedures** should be considered in the setting of failed prior arthroscopic stabilization procedures and large bony defects.
  - ▫ Failure of arthroscopic Bankart repairs[10]
    - 79% have inverted pear-shaped bony Bankart lesions.
    - 21% have engaging Hill-Sachs lesions.
  - ▫ Bony involvement
    - Osseous glenoid defects greater than 21% of the width leads to a significant increase in shoulder instability with soft-tissue procedures alone and is an indication for bony reconstructive procedures during Bankart repairs.[11]
    - Glenoid reconstructive options
      - ○ Latarjet procedure (coracoid transfer)
      - ○ Iliac crest bone graft
  - ▫ A diagnostic arthroscopy should be considered even when open intervention is planned. Seventy-three percent of patients undergoing Latarjet glenoid reconstruction have additional pathology including superior labral anterior-posterior (SLAP) tears, loose bodies, chondral damage, and rotator cuff tears.[12]

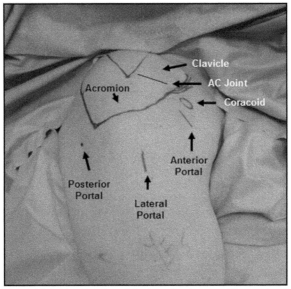

Figure 14-6. Identification of the bony landmarks with associated arthroscopic portal placement.

SURGICAL ANATOMY

Despite the evolution of arthroscopy in the management of shoulder instability, an understanding of the underlying anatomy is critical to minimize complications and re-establish the damaged structures.

Arthroscopy

- Identification of the bony landmarks is necessary for accurate portal placement (Figure 14-6).
- Proper portal placement allows for adequate visualization of the glenohumeral joint and provides working access for instrumentation (Figure 14-7).

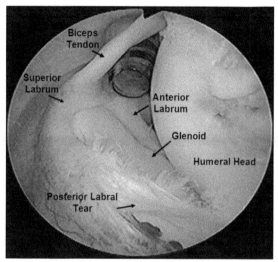

Figure 14-7. Arthroscopic view from the posterior portal illustrating the anatomy of the glenohumeral joint. Note the tear of the posterior labrum. The anterior portal also is visualized as the cannula adjacent to the biceps tendon.

- The joint capsule forms ligamentous condensations including the SGHL, MGHL, and anterior and posterior band of the IGHL that are key contributors to shoulder stability.
- The insertion of the glenohumeral ligament on the humerus also is associated with shoulder instability and should be identified during arthroscopy (Figure 14-8).

Open Procedures

- Bony landmarks are utilized and a deltopectoral incision is made based on coracoid process

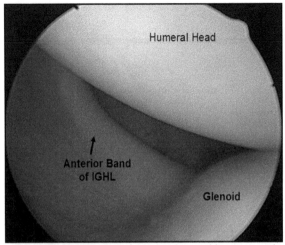

Figure 14-8. The insertion of the glenohumeral ligament on the humerus is inspected to rule out avulsion injuries that can lead to instability. The anterior band of the inferior glenohumeral ligament (IGHL) is identified.

proximally and along the deltopectoral groove distally (Figure 14-9).

- The deltopectoral groove is identified; the cephalic vein is evident within the interval (Figure 14-10).
- Retraction within the deltopectoral interval allows visualization of the subscapularis muscle, the biceps tendon within the bicipital groove, and the greater tuberosity (Figure 14-11).
- This approach is appropriate for Latarjet, iliac crest bone graft, and capsular shift procedures.

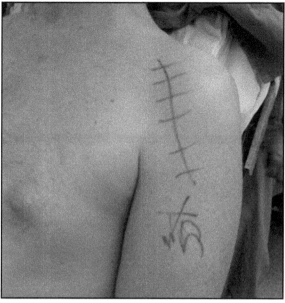

Figure 14-9. The coracoid is identified proximally and the skin incision is based along the deltopectoral groove distally. A more vertically based incision from the coracoid process to the axilla may be utilized for Latarjet and capsular shift type procedures.

PROCEDURES

- An examination is performed under anesthesia and the direction of the instability is assessed. Comparison is made to examination of the normal shoulder. Range of motion is documented.
- Arthroscopic stabilization
  - Depending on surgeon preference, the patient may be positioned either in the beach chair or lateral decubitus position.

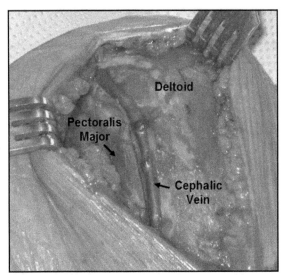

Figure 14-10. The cephalic vein lies in the interval between the deltoid and pectoralis major muscles.

- □ The posterior portal is established and diagnostic arthroscopy of the glenohumeral joint performed. Then, under direct visualization, 2 anterior portals are created in preparation for an anterior labral repair.
- □ A similar technique is used for posterior instability, during which the anterior portal is placed first.
- □ An 18-gauge spinal needle is placed initially to optimize the trajectory of the portal.
- □ Diagnostic arthroscopy is performed using standard anterior and posterior portals. The joint is inspected. Particular attention is paid to the capsule, labrum, and glenoid because the majority of the pathology involves these tissues.

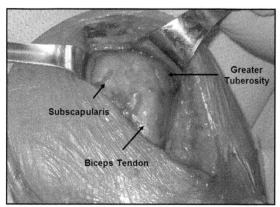

Figure 14-11. Retraction within the deltopectoral interval allows for visualization of the subscapularis muscle, biceps tendon within the bicipital groove, and the greater tuberosity.

- □ After the underlying pathology is identified, attention is directed toward repair (Figure 14-12).
- □ A drill guide is used for placement of the suture anchors (Figure 14-13).
- □ After anchor placement, the suture is passed through the damaged capsulolabral tissue (Figure 14-14).
- □ The sutures are tied, securing the labrum to the native footprint (Figure 14-15).
- Open stabilization
  - □ Many options exist for anterior stabilization via a deltopectoral approach:
    - Latarjet
    - Iliac crest bone graft
    - Allograft glenoid reconstruction
    - Capsular shift
    - Capsular allograft/autograft reconstruction

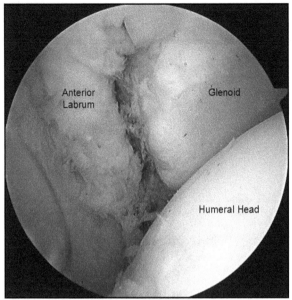

Figure 14-12. Arthroscopic visualization from the anterior portal reveals detachment of the anterior labrum from the glenoid.

- □ Latarjet reconstruction is a viable initial option, as the subscapularis is not detached but rather the intramuscular interval is utilized.
- □ Iliac crest bone graft can be used in situations involving large defects or failed prior bony procedures.
  - After detachment of the subscapularis and identification of the underlying capsule, the defect on the glenoid is identified.

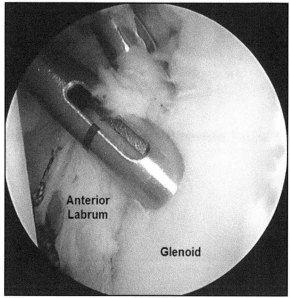

Figure 14-13. A drill guide is placed on the periphery of the glenoid allowing for placement on suture anchors.

- Depending on surgeon preference, the bony allograft or autograft is contoured to fit the glenoid defect.
- The bone is held in place with temporary Kirschner wires.
- Screw fixation provides stability while the graft is incorporated (Figure 14-16).
- The capsule is reapproximated and the subscapularis repaired.

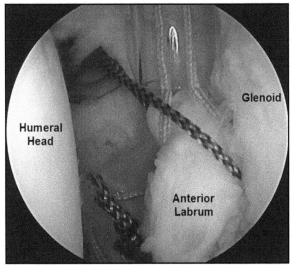

Figure 14-14. The sutures are placed through the damaged capsule and labrum.

REHABILITATION[13]

Arthroscopic Anterior Stabilization

- Weeks 0 to 6: The shoulder is immobilized in a sling; the arm is maintained in internal rotation. Active and passive range of motion of the wrist, elbow, and hand are performed.
- Weeks 4 to 6: Passive range of motion of the shoulder may be started when approved by the surgeon.
- Weeks 6 to 7: Full active range of motion begins. Gradual (external rotation passive range of motion) begins at lower angles (less than 20 degrees of abduction); progressive increases in abduction

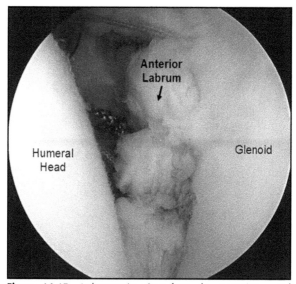

Figure 14-15. Arthroscopic view from the posterior portal demonstrating final repair of the anterior labral tear.

are performed at the discretion of the surgeon. No weight lifting is allowed. The patient is weaned from the sling.

- Weeks 8 to 12: Progressive strengthening and passive range of motion are performed.
- Weeks 12+: Continued strengthening is followed by transition to sport-specific activities.
- Criteria for return to play:
  - ☐ Surgeon clearance
  - ☐ Pain-free range of motion
  - ☐ Strength comparable to noninjured arm

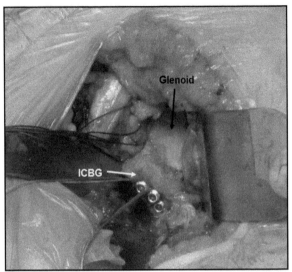

Figure 14-16. Iliac crest bone graft (ICBG) reconstruction of the anterior glenoid. Screw fixation provides stability while the graft heals to the glenoid.

Open Anterior Shoulder Stabilization

- Weeks 0 to 2: The arm is immobilized in a sling. Therapy involves passive range of motion with forward flexion limited to 90 degrees, external rotation to 0 degrees, and internal rotation to 45 degrees at 30 degrees of abduction. Active and passive range of motion of the wrist, elbow, and hand are performed.
- Weeks 2 to 4: Sling immobilization continues. Passive range of motion progresses to full forward flexion, full internal rotation, and 30 degrees of external rotation.

- Weeks 4 to 6: The patient is weaned from the sling as directed per surgeon. Progression to full active range of motion follows.
- Weeks 6 to 10: Progression to full passive range of motion, including external rotation, is directed. Strengthening begins.
- Weeks 10 to 16: Continued strengthening follows with transition to sport-specific activities.

Posterior Stabilization

- Weeks 0 to 4: The shoulder is immobilized in a sling, positioning the shoulder with 30 degrees of abduction and 15 degrees of external rotation. No flexion is allowed. Active and passive range of motion of the wrist, elbow, and hand are performed. Internal rotation exercises are avoided.
- Weeks 4 of 6: The patient is weaned from the sling and internal rotation is advanced based on surgeon recommendations. Active assisted range of motion with pulleys and active range of motion with abduction to 90 degrees, external rotation to 90 degrees, and internal rotation to 35 degrees are performed. Gentle capsular stretching is used as indicated.
- Weeks 6 to 12: Active assisted and active range of motion are directed as tolerated in all planes except for internal rotation, which is limited to 40 degrees. Strengthening begins.
- Weeks 12 to 18: Progressive strengthening and neuromuscular development are emphasized.
- Weeks 19+: Continued strengthening follows with transition to sport-specific activities.

Outcomes

Outcomes following Bankart repair must be considered in the context of several factors: the type of repair (open versus arthroscopic), patient factors (gender, athletic versus non-athletic, single versus multiple dislocations), sport (contact versus noncontact), and presence or absence of glenoid bone loss. Furthermore, outcomes such as range of motion, return to activities, recurrence of dislocation, and pain must be considered with respect to goals of individual patients. Grumet, Bach, and Provencher[14] summarize the past 15 years of outcomes following surgical stabilization.

Potential Complications

- Recurrent instability
- Nerve injury (axillary or musculocutaneous nerves)
- Infection
- Stiffness
- Pain
- Arthritis

References

1. Beighton P, Solomon L, Soskolne CL. Articular mobility in an African population. *Ann Rheum Dis*. 1973;32:413-418.
2. Itoi E, Hatakeyama Y, Sato T, et al. Immobilization in external rotation after shoulder dislocation reduces the risk of recurrence. A randomized controlled trial. *J Bone Joint Surg Am*. 2007;89(10):2124-2131.
3. Hovelius L, Augustini BG, Fredin H, Johansson O, Norlin R, Thorling J. Primary anterior dislocation of the shoulder in young patients. A ten-year prospective study. *J Bone Joint Surg Am*. 1996;78(11):1677-1684.

4. Hovelius L, Olofsson A, Sandström B, et al. Nonoperative treatment of primary anterior shoulder dislocation in patients forty years of age and younger: a prospective twenty-five-year follow-up. *J Bone Joint Surg Am.* 2008;90(5):945-952.

5. Burkhead WZ Jr, Rockwood CA Jr. Treatment of instability of the shoulder with an exercise program. *J Bone Joint Surg Am.* 1992;74(6):890-896.

6. Taylor DC, Arciero RA. Pathologic changes associated with shoulder dislocations. Arthroscopic and physical examination findings in first-time, traumatic anterior dislocations. *Am J Sports Med.* 1997;25(3):306-311.

7. Calandra JJ, Baker CL, Uribe J. The incidence of Hill-Sachs lesions in initial anterior shoulder dislocations. *Arthroscopy.* 1989;5(4):254-257.

8. Kirkley A, Griffin S, Richards C, Miniaci A, Mohtadi N. Prospective randomized clinical trial comparing the effectiveness of immediate arthroscopic stabilization versus immobilization and rehabilitation in first traumatic anterior dislocations of the shoulder. *Arthroscopy.* 1999;15(5):507-514.

9. Brophy RH, Marx RG. The treatment of traumatic anterior instability of the shoulder: nonoperative and surgical treatment. *Arthroscopy.* 2009;25(3):298-304. Review.

10. Burkhart SS, De Beer JF. Traumatic glenohumeral bone defects and their relationship to failure of arthroscopic Bankart repairs: significance of the inverted-pear glenoid and the humeral engaging Hill-Sachs lesion. *Arthroscopy.* 2000;16(7):677-694.

11. Itoi E, Lee SB, Berglund LJ, Berge LL, An KN. The effect of a glenoid defect on anteroinferior stability of the shoulder after Bankart repair: a cadaveric study. *J Bone Joint Surg Am.* 2000;82(1):35-46.

12. Arrigoni P, Huberty D, Brady PC, Weber IC, Burkhart SS. The value of arthroscopy before an open modified latarjet reconstruction. *Arthroscopy.* 2008;24(5):514-519.

13. Rehabilitation protocols adapted from Harvard Shoulder Service/Brigham and Women's Hospital Department of Rehabilitation Services. www.bosshin.com. Accessed March 9, 2011.

14. Grumet R, Bach B Jr, Provencher M. Arthroscopic stabilization for first-time versus recurrent shoulder instability. *Arthroscopy.* 2010;26(2):239-248.

Relevant Review Articles

Millett PJ, Clavert P, Hatch GFR, Warner JJP. Recurrent posterior shoulder instability. *J Am Acad Orthop Surg.* 2006;14(8):464-476.

Millett PJ, Clavert P, Warner JJP. Arthroscopic management of anterior, posterior, and multidirectional shoulder instability: pearls and pitfalls. *Arthroscopy.* 2003;19 (Suppl 1):86-93.

APPENDIX

SHOULDER IMPINGEMENT EXAMINATION
Neer Sign
The finding is pathologic for subacromial impingement if pain is felt while the fully pronated arm is passively flexed forward above 90 degrees with a fixed scapula.

Hawkins-Kennedy Test
The result is pathologic for subacromial impingement or rotator cuff tendinitis if pain is felt when arm is forcefully internally rotated while in 90 degrees (also known as Hawkins sign or Hawkins test).

Neer Impingement Test
The finding is positive when pain caused by the Neer sign maneuver described above is alleviated (ie, disappears) with a selective injection of local anesthetic into the subacromial space.

ROTATOR CUFF STRENGTH TESTS
Supraspinatus
Drop Arm Sign
The finding is pathologic for supraspinatus insufficiency if the patient cannot hold the passively abducted arm in place or if the arm cannot be lowered slowly without dropping.

Rohde RS, Millett PJ, eds.
Evaluation and Management of Common Upper Extremity Disorders: A Practical Handbook (pp 271-276).
© 2011 Taylor & Francis Group.

Empty Can Test

This is a strength test for the supraspinatus with the internally rotated arm ("thumb down") held against resistance in 90-degree abduction in the plane of the scapula.

Subscapularis

Lift-Off Test

The result is pathologic for subscapularis insufficiency if a passively maximally internally rotated arm cannot be held elevated from the back. If elevation is possible, hand-back distance can be measured and compared to that of the contralateral arm. In the modified lift-off test, the arm is positioned off the back and the patient is instructed to hold it there. If the arm falls back or the patient cannot maintain the position, the test result is considered positive.

Belly Press Test

In this strength test for the subscapularis, the patient places the hand on the abdomen and resists the examiner's attempts to externally rotate the arm. Insufficiency is demonstrated if the elbow migrates dorsally and the wrist flexes while the patient is resisting. With a postive test result (ie, in cases of complete subscapularis tear) the arm cannot be maintained on the stomach with any degree of force.

Infraspinatus

External Rotation

This is a strength test to evaluate the infraspinatus and teres minor, performed by having the patient provide external rotation against resistance with the arm at the side and the elbow at 90-degree flexion. An external rotation lag sign is seen when the passively externally rotated arm falls back. This is due to insufficiency of the infraspinatus.

Teres Minor
Hornblower's Sign
The finding is pathologic for infraspinatus and teres minor insufficiency if external rotation weakness or lag occurs at 90-degree abduction in the scapular plane or if the patient's elbow rises above hand level when the hand is raised to the mouth.

Shoulder Instability Examination
Anterior Instability
Fulcrum Test
This test is performed supine with the patient's body as counterweight, the table edge as the fulcrum, and the arm as the lever. The shoulder is in 90-degree abduction and external rotation. The test is positive if progressive external rotation causes apprehensive reaction or instability.

Fowler's Sign/Relocation Test
This is an addition to the fulcrum test and is performed by pushing posteriorly on the proximal humerus. The test result is positive if more external rotation can be applied before re-emergence of an apprehension sign.

Anterior Apprehension Test
This test is performed with the examiner's fingers over the humeral head and the thumb pushing the humeral head from behind and externally rotating the patient's arm in abducted position. The finding is positive if progressive external rotation causes apprehensive reaction or instability.

Load and Shift Test

This test is performed by the examiner stabilizing the shoulder girdle with one hand on the shoulder and scapula and the other hand grasping the humeral head. The humerus is loaded into the glenoid centrally and translated anteriorly, posteriorly, and inferiorly. As the stress applied is increased, the humeral head may be felt to ride up and/or over the glenoid rim. Examination should be performed in upright and supine positions. The test result is positive if translation can be felt.

Posterior Instability

Posterior Apprehension Test

This test is performed by pushing the flexed and adducted arm posteriorly. The test result is positive if the maneuver causes apprehensive reaction or instability.

Load and Shift Test

This test is described under Anterior Instability.

Inferior Laxity

Inferior Apprehension Test

The examiner supports the 90-degree abducted arm with one hand. With the other hand, the examiner tries to invoke an inferior subluxation by applying pressure downward on the patient's upper arm.

Inferior Sulcus Test

This test is performed with the patient sitting or standing and the shoulder in neutral position. Applying inferior traction, the examiner watches for dimpling of the skin below the acromion and palpates potential widening of the subacromial space. The test result is positive if the humeral head moves more than 1 cm.

Biceps Tendon Examination
Yergason's Test
This test, designed to assess for pathology in the long head of the biceps tendon in its sheath, is performed by the patient trying to supinate against resistance while the examiner holds the patient's arms at the wrists. The patient's elbow is flexed 90 degrees and the forearms are pronated. The test result is positive if pain is located in the bicipital groove.

Speed's Test
This test, designed to assess for pathology in the long head of the biceps tendon in its groove, is performed by the examiner resisting humeral forward flexion. The patient's elbow is extended, the forearm supinated, and the humerus elevated to 60 degrees. The test result is positive if pain is located in the bicipital groove.

Ludington's Test
Designed to identify rupture of the tendon of the long biceps head, this test is performed by the seated patient placing the hands behind the head with interlocked fingers. The patient contracts and relaxes the biceps while the examiner palpates the tendon of the long biceps head. The test result is positive if the examiner cannot feel the biceps tendon.

SLAP Lesion Tests
Active Compression Test or O'Brien's Test
This test is designed to assess acromioclavicular joint and labral pathology. The patient's shoulder is flexed 90 degrees, with the elbows fully extended and

arms adducted 10 to 15 degrees medial to the saggital plane. The arms are maximally internally rotated and the patient resists the examiner's downward force. The procedure is repeated in supination. The test result is positive if pain is provoked by the first maneuver and reduced by the second one.

SLAPrehension Test

This test is designed to assess labral pathology. The patient's arm is flexed 90 degrees across the chest, with the elbows fully extended and forearms pronated. The procedure is repeated in supination. The test result is positive if pain and/or a click is provoked in the area of the bicipital groove in pronation and pain is reduced in supination.

FINANCIAL DISCLOSURES

Dr. Robert E. Boykin has no financial or proprietary interest in the materials presented herein.

Dr. Sepp Braun has no financial or proprietary interest in the materials presented herein.

Dr. Michael Darowish has no financial or proprietary interest in the materials presented herein.

Dr. Christopher B. Dewing has no financial or proprietary interest in the materials presented herein.

Dr. Florian Elser was an Arthrex research fellow (Steadman Hawkins Resarch Foundation) in 2008-2009.

Dr. David C. Gerhardt has no financial or proprietary interest in the materials presented herein.

Dr. Reuben Gobezie is a consultant for Arthrex Inc and Tornier, and he receives research funding from both of these entities.

Dr. Danny P. Goel has no financial or proprietary interest in the materials presented herein.

Dr. Robert R. L. Gray has no financial or proprietary interest in the materials presented herein.

Dr. James J. Guerra is a consultant for Arthrex Inc.

Mr. Hinrich J. D. Heuer has no financial or proprietary interest in the materials presented herein.

Dr. Christopher J. Lenarz has no financial or proprietary interest in the materials presented herein.

Dr. Kimberly Mezera has no financial or proprietary interest in the materials presented herein.

Dr. Peter J. Millett is a consultant for and receives royalties from Arthrex Inc. He is also an investor of Game Ready.

Dr. Ryan G. Miyamoto has no financial or proprietary interest in the materials presented herein.

Dr. Charles J. Petit has no financial or proprietary interest in the materials presented herein.

Dr. Brent A. Ponce has no financial or proprietary interest in the materials presented herein.

Dr. Rachel S. Rohde has no financial or proprietary interest in the materials presented herein.

Dr. James R. Romanowski has no financial or proprietary interest in the materials presented herein.

Dr. Gregory V. Sobol has no financial or proprietary interest in the materials presented herein.

Dr. Peter Tang has no financial or proprietary interest in the materials presented herein.

Dr. Walter W. Virkus has no financial or proprietary interest in the materials presented herein.

Dr. Jon J. P. Warner receives royalties from Zimmer Co for a shoulder prosthesis.

Dr. Trent J. Wilson has no financial or proprietary interest in the materials presented herein.

Dr. Jennifer Moriatis Wolf is the Elsevier updates editor, *Journal of Hand Surgery* deputy editor, and Vindico Medical Education hand module editor. She receives funding from the Orthopaedic Research and Education Foundation and American Foundation for Surgery of the Hand.

INDEX